17 WISE WAYS TO DAILY OUTSMART DIABETES

KENNETH R. ELLIS, M.S.
with Deb Ellis, Contributor

DISCLAIMER: The information in this book should not replace consultations with qualified healthcare professionals to meet your individual medical needs.

ISBN: 9798863494463 (paperback, 2nd edition)
    9798864594926 (hardback, 1st edition)
    9798863494463 (ebook)

Also by Kenneth R. Ellis

The Way of Wisdom for Health:
Optimism, Kindness, Motivation, Movement,
Nutrition, and Stress Control

The Way of Wisdom for Diabetes:
Cope with Stress, Move More, Lose Weight and
Keep Hope Alive

Subscribe to the
Wisdom for Diabetes YouTube Channel
www.wisdomfordiabetes.org

CONTENTS

PART 1: 17 WISE WAYS TO DAILY OUTSMART DIABETES

PART 2: COMMON SENSE GUIDELINES FOR LIVING WELL WITH DIABETES

Part 1
17 Wise Ways to Daily Outsmart Diabetes

Introduction

A s a man steps off the curb and begins to walk across the street, a car comes screeching around the corner. The car is coming straight toward the man. He picks up his pace, trying to hurry across the street. The car changes lanes and comes straight toward him. So, he turns around to go back, but the car changes lanes too. The car is so close, and the man is so scared that he freezes. The car swerves at the last moment to miss the man and screeches to a stop. The window comes down. The driver is a squirrel who says, "See, it's not as easy as it looks, is it?"

There may have been a time when you thought someone should handle some stressful situation better. Then, after experiencing something similar, you find out that "it's not as easy as it looks." Having a similar experience is necessary to understand how it feels.

When I look at people who struggle with their diabetes to control their blood sugars, I know from my experience that "it's not as easy as it looks." I want to make suggestions, tips, and ideas from my experience and research. We need the motivation to do the right things, which we can build with God's wisdom! As you continue to read this book, you will notice how God's wisdom intricately applies to life's situations and how that wisdom directly relates to our health. What I experience each day illustrates how wisdom can apply. When I get up in the morning, blood sugar is first on my mind. What is my blood glucose level? Is it high, low, or is it just right? I check my blood first thing in the morning. Then throughout the day, those thoughts stay with me. After eating lunch, I wonder if I took enough insulin for the carbohydrates I ate. I check my blood sugar if I'm not wearing my continuous glucose monitor sensor. Multiple times each day, I check my blood glucose, think about the amount of exercise I'm getting and the number of grams of carbohydrates I'm eating.

I do this to ensure I get the proper balance of food, activity, and insulin to maintain blood sugar levels as close to normal as possible. Do I succeed? Most of the time. You may think what an annoyance, nuisance, or hassle! Is that any way to live a life? Yes, it is because to think this way is the "way of wisdom." Proverbs 4:23 states, *"Be careful what you think, because your thoughts run your life."* God's wisdom states, *"Pleasant words are like honey. They are sweet to the spirit and bring healing to the body"* (Proverbs 16:24).

If you need to think about your health, what you eat, and how many steps you take, start. It is the "way of wisdom" or "the skill for living." *"A good person gives life to others; the wise person teaches others how to live… Keep their words in mind forever as though you had them tied around your neck. They will guide you when you walk. They will guard you when you sleep. They will speak to you when you are awake"* (Proverbs 11:30, 6:21-22 NCV).

Wisdom's Value—The Skill for Living

"When you walk, they will guide you; when you sleep, they will watch over you; when you awake, they will speak to you." (Proverbs 6:22).

The foundation for these outsmarting strategies is the way of wisdom (skill for living), God's wisdom. Success and victory come from God's wisdom. *"For the LORD gives wisdom; from his mouth come knowledge and understanding. He holds success in store for the upright"* (Proverbs 2:6-7). We all have available to us God's wisdom which is more precious than rubies. *"She is more precious than rubies; nothing you desire can compare with her"* (Proverbs 3:15). As you read through these strategies, you will see how vital and valuable the resource of wisdom is. It could be called the common-sense approach that is not so common.

Diabetes Management application: By doing the following 17 prime activities, you'll keep your safety harness on. Instead of letting diabetes do its devastating work in the background of your life, destroying your health, you will keep in control. So, let's start our day with seven vital guidelines.

CHAPTER ONE

Staying in Control in the Morning

#1   Keep Learning.

Ignorance is not bliss. When I went to see my Endocrinologist recently, I told him since I'm 69, I decided to try two new things. The first one was to donate blood. I tried to donate forty years ago but was not accepted since I had Type 1 Diabetes. But this time, I was accepted as long as I didn't have current diabetes complications and was in stable control. So my wife and I gave. And after doing so, I had a wonderful feeling about the good it would do.

The second thing I decided to do was look at the best-seller book list on Amazon for books under the category of Diabetes. When I saw the Diabetes Code was number 1, I decided to buy it. What a wise decision that was.

It is good to start the day knowing what Diabetes is. The better we understand, the better our choices will be. Instead of assuming what we need to do, we can know what to do. For example, someone asked me, since I have Type 1 Diabetes, when I would become Type 2. The fact is I will never become Type 2. Both types of Diabetes have similar lifestyles with meal plans and exercise but are dissimilar in many ways, like medications available for use. Both can use an effective therapy, but the results can reverse Type 2 Diabetes. Type 1s can use it to lose weight and cause their bodies to be more sensitive to insulin, making less needed. What is this therapy I discovered? Fasting and I found it in the information author and medical doctor Jason Fung wrote in the Diabetes Code.

The essential difference between the two types of Diabetes is the beta cells available in the pancreas to produce insulin. Type 1 is an autoimmune disease in which the body attacks and destroys the insulin-producing beta cells. Type 2 is a disease in which the beta cells keep producing to the point of stuffing the cells with glucose. That is how there becomes insulin resistance. Instead of being stored as glycogen, the body stores the excess glucose as fat. When fasting for sixteen hours, the body, after fourteen hours, uses the stored glucose, which is glycogen, and then converts to fat as its energy source. This means that the body begins to lose weight. So, it is imperative with either type to keep blood glucose as close to the normal range as possible and know that carbohydrates profoundly impact blood glucose levels and insulin production in people with Type 2 Diabetes. I give more information on metabolism with the fourth wise way of timing.

Watch: To view an explanation of how insulin moves glucose into cells, go to "Insulin, Glucose and You" at https://www.youtube.com/watch?v=jqP9JmS_sKo.

After knowing what Diabetes is, we need a plan to outsmart it daily! Almost everyone has a routine in the morning, but is it best for your health?

#2 Have a health routine—a plan.

"Proper Prior Planning Prevents Pitifully Poor Performance. People Don't Plan to Fail, They Fail to Plan. Planning the Best Decisions Ahead of Time: Diligence"

"The wisdom of the prudent is to give thought to their ways, but the folly of fools is deception" (Proverbs 14:8).

"Sluggards do not plow in season; so at harvest time they look but find nothing" (Proverbs 20:4).

"The plans of the diligent lead to profit as surely as haste leads to poverty" (Proverbs 21:5).

Biblically, the basic meaning of diligence is planning.

People get out of bed in the morning and usually visit the restroom. What follows among people differs. Some have the simple habit of making their bed. Making your bed first thing in the morning is good, but there is a plan that is much more beneficial for those with diabetes!

Planning keeps you free to control your diabetes. The desire to go back and do things differently happens in many situations. For example, have you ever locked your car and looked in to see your keys sitting on the seat? Even worse, what if you got locked into an ATM service room? A recent news headline was "Texas Police Make Odd Withdrawal from ATM: A Man Who Was Trapped Inside."[1] A contractor, who was changing the lock on the service room of an ATM, realized he had locked himself in the room. Unfortunately, he couldn't call anyone for help because he had left his cell phone in his truck.

What was he to do? He became very creative. People started receiving more than cash and a receipt at the ATM. They also got a handwritten note with their receipt — "Please Help. I'm stuck in here, and I don't have my phone. Please call my boss. At 210..." He did this for about two hours until one person finally took the message and called the police. "This is just a prank" is what most people thought, including the police, until someone behind the screen answered them. They broke the door down and freed the desperate man. A police officer said, "We have a once-in-a-lifetime situation that you'll probably never see or hear about again."

What lessons can we learn from this? First, giving thought to health is so important! How many times will I check my blood sugar today? Or how many steps will I take? How many calories will I eat, especially carbohydrates, since they directly impact my blood sugar levels? These are the things to think about first thing in the morning! The way of God's wisdom teaches the importance of planning, of not getting in a hurry, of not having to go back and do things differently. *"The plans of the diligent lead to profit as surely as haste leads to poverty"* (Proverbs 21: 5). *"Enthusiasm without knowledge is not good. If you act too quickly, you might make a mistake"* (Proverbs 19: 2). We all need to plan our days, build healthy habits, and to think before doing!

Watch: "Police Withdraw Man Trapped In Bank ATM" at https://www.youtube.com/watch?v=DDU7ibWTX9U.

#3 Check your blood glucose level first thing in the morning!

Pricking your fingers hurts! So, why do it? (You experience less pain by pricking on the side of your finger, not the pad. Use a good lancet device like a "CareTouch," too.) Discovering your blood glucose will give you the information to make the best decision. What if you wake up with an elevated blood glucose of 185 or even 264? What should you do? Should you go ahead and eat breakfast? No, take a leisure walk instead, or avoid carbs for breakfast. What caused this? What was my blood glucose last night before going to bed? Do I have a cold starting? Did I eat a snack last night? Have relationship conflicts or financial stress? All these could be factors that cause elevated blood glucose in the morning. Where should your blood glucose be during the day? Here are some guidelines compared to normal numbers for those without diabetes.

Nighttime fasting and before breakfast: 70–130 mg/dl
Normal is less than 100 mg/dl
Before lunch, supper, and snacks: 70–130 mg/dl
Two hours after starting meals: 160 mg/dl or less
Normal is less than 140 mg/dl
Bedtime: 90–150 mg/dl
Normal is less than 120 mg/dl
http://www.joslin.org/docs/Pharm_Guideline_Graded.pdf

Many people have the good habit of checking their blood glucose in the morning—and then they are through checking for the day! However, research indicates that checking yourself more often than once daily will build greater self-management confidence and better glucose numbers. From this research, the A1c test results fell more than one point—7.3 to 6.2. (For more information on this topic, read pp. 31-37 in my book "The Way of Wisdom for Diabetes.")

#4 Mimic God's design of the body with timing—making the right time your habit.

"Timing Is (Almost) Everything"

Wisdom's way teaches the importance of timing:

"Anyone who refuses to work doesn't plow in the right season. When he looks for a crop at harvest time, he doesn't find it." (Proverbs 20:4 NIrV).

"A person finds joy in giving an apt reply—and how good is a timely word!" (Proverbs 15:23)

Since carbohydrates affect blood glucose, take your insulin before breakfast or any meal (unless your blood glucose is below 70, then take it after the meal). Novolog and Humalog become active within fifteen to twenty minutes. So, if you wake up at 163, take your insulin, walk and then eat breakfast, you could have low blood glucose. This happened with a friend of mine, and before he could get to breakfast, he was 38 mg/dl.

Mimic God's design of the body.

"We are fearfully and wonderfully made" (Psalm 139:14). God's wisdom teachings are for the health of one's whole body. *"Turn your ear to my words...for they are life to those who find them and health to one's whole body"* (Proverbs 4:20, 22). The Proverbs teaches principles like this one. *"Finish your outdoor work and get your fields ready; after that, build your house"* (Proverbs 24:27). The proverb teaches an important sequence concerning

a person's financial welfare. If a person doesn't have the fields ready, there will not be a harvest for food to eat on the table. Building a house will not sustain a person with the nourishment needed. So, get your fields ready, so there can be a harvest and then have resources to build a house. A sequence of priority steps is needed for physical health too. So walk, eat, check blood glucose, take medications, and do so at just the right time! "You've got to be kidding?" No, we've already seen the importance of a sequence when starting the day.

We see a sequence in God's design of the body when we eat. What happens when we eat carbohydrates? Glucose is the result. First, the body transports Glucose with blood into the small intestine. Then, a step-by-step process begins to metabolize the Glucose for energy. In a sense, the body is counting the carbs you eat and initially responds by releasing stored-up insulin in secretory vesicles in the pancreas. Then it begins to manufacture the exact amount of insulin needed with the pancreas' beta cells.

Do you know you have some tiny but priceless islands? The Pancreas' Islets of Langerhans (about 1 million of them) are the priceless islands. They are priceless because, within each one, you have about two thousand beta cells and alpha cells (producing the hormone glucagon). Within the beta cells, the hormone insulin is manufactured in a multi-step process; the word insulin is from a Latin root word meaning island. And insulin is produced in the Islets of Langerhans. "These are capable of measuring the blood glucose level within seconds with an accuracy to within 2 mg/dl (0.1 mmol/1) to determine the quantity of insulin needed," writes Dr. Richard Beaser of the Joslin Diabetes

Center.[2] Especially when we eat carbohydrates, glucose levels rise. Stored insulin then deploys rapidly, which is called phase 1 insulin release. Unfortunately, most people with Type 2 diabetes have an impaired phase 1 release of insulin. This can cause a high blood glucose reading after a meal and a low hypoglycemic episode several hours later with too much insulin in circulation.

Insulin is a multifaceted hormone capable of doing several functions, and here are some of them. Insulin aids glucose entry into cells for energy storage and heat production. Since its discovery 100 years ago, this has been the focus of insulin. When Banting and Best discovered insulin, doctors used it for patients needing glucose control. And even the term "diabetes (siphon Greek), mellitus (sweet Latin)" evokes the "honey urine that attracts ants" idea recognized since antiquity but first documented by Thomas Willis in 1674. With the use of insulin, patients and healthcare providers focus on Blood sugar control to prevent complications. This has been my focus as a person with Type 1 Diabetes for about sixty-three years, and it brings life instead of death for Type 1s.

People newly diagnosed with diabetes can be confused about what to eat and what not to eat. One man said, *"My doctor told me about the importance of a healthy meal plan, which— as near as I can tell—means I'm only allowed to eat birdseed all day."* At one time, it was almost that bad. Before 1921, people took drastic measures to continue to breathe with no quality of life. In 1919, Dr. Frederick Allen published Total Dietary Regulation in the Treatment of Diabetes, citing detailed case records of 76 of the 100 diabetes patients he observed—called Type 1 patients today! His treatment for them was to start with an extremely low-carbohydrate diet and gradually increase to the renal threshold, or the level of blood glucose above which the kidneys fail to reabsorb—and thus spill—glucose into the urine. The renal threshold is about 180 mg/dl. What this meant for most people was living on a diet plan or "starvation therapy" of very little food per day. They virtually eliminated carbs from their diet. So we can summarize the treatment as eat less, be hungrier!

Dr. Banting was a surgeon during World War 1. While in the battle zone, shrapnel wounded his right forearm. They removed it and applied a tourniquet above his elbow. He then continued to work on the injured for seventeen hours. This is the kind of character he had!

After his time in World War 1, he became a demonstrator in surgery and anatomy at the University of Western Ontario. In this role, he had to talk to medical students about the pancreas, which led him to read about the islets of Langerhans in a medical journal. His idea was to extract a substance from the islets, later known as insulin, using the lab at Toronto University. He and a graduate assistant, Charles Best, used lab dogs, dog pound dogs, and even strays that summer for their experiments. Dr. Frederick Banting and Charles Best tied off the pancreas duct in dogs and discovered insulin on July 27, 1921.

Dr. Allen returns from Toronto after visiting Dr. Banting to his treatment clinic, and this is what happened. "Diabetics who had not been out of bed for weeks began to trail weakly about, clinging to walls and furniture. It was a resurrection. When he appeared through the open doorway, he caught the full beseeching of a hundred pairs of eyes," writes nurse Margate

Kienast. His voice curiously mingled concern for his patients with excitement that he tried his best not to betray. "I think," he said, "I think we have something for you." So what became the treatment and management of Type 1 & 2 diabetes for decades? Insulin! Now we see these ways to manage Type 2 diabetes—improved diet, regular exercise, healthy weight, medications to control blood sugar, and self-management through lifestyle. But these do not address the core issue of Type 2 Diabetes, which we will look at in a few pages.

Here is another function of insulin. Insulin enhances the process by which cells make proteins and cell growth. Insulin increases protein synthesis because insulin is one of the ana-bolic (growth and building) hormones along with growth hor-mone in the body. Insulin builds! Its main action is "opening" the cells so glucose can enter. Insulin also promotes protein synthesis by aiding the amino acids' entry into cells. Amino acids are molecules that combine to form proteins. Amino acids and proteins are the building blocks of life.[3]

But too much insulin affects people with insulin resistance and eventually Type 2 Diabetes. The liver stockpiles glucose into glycogen. But the liver has its limits for glycogen storage. Once that limit is reached, the overflow in glucose triggers another insulin function. It starts the liver with the excess glucose into fat through de novo lipogenesis (DNL). De novo (from new) and lipogenesis (making new fat), so De novo lipogenesis means "to make new fat." Insulin turns excess glucose into new fat in the form of triglyceride molecules. This new fat is stored in fat cells that the body can use for energy.

Insulin Resistance and Hyperinsulinemia occur when the

cells are already full of glucose and the glucose-to-fat conversion starts. According to Dr. Jason Fung, this results in more stored fat or fatty liver. Insulin will also reduce fat movement. So where do you want to move fat? Out of the organs and fat around organs.[4]

Your body also can self-heal by not trying to eat when you are ill. In other words, your body goes into a fasting state. A fasting state can be healthy for losing weight and cutting back on the need for more insulin.

Jesus fasted. *"After fasting forty days and forty nights, he was hungry"* (Matthew 4:2). Jesus was very weak, and Satan knew he was. This is when he tempted him by saying to turn stones into bread. But Jesus demonstrated that even in his condition, he could resist the temptation to use his powers in a self-centered way. But the point is Jesus fasted. Here is what other noteworthy people from history have said about fasting. "Instead of using medicine, better fast today," said Plutarch. "I fast for greater physical and mental efficiency," said Plato. Benjamin Franklin wrote, "The best of all medicines is resting and fasting." "Everyone has a doctor in him; we just have to help him in his work. The natural healing force within each one of us is the greatest force in getting well...to eat when you are sick, is to feed your sickness," said Hippocrates.

To give you the full perspective on insulin's primary function to analyze, here is the traditional explanation. "Produced in the pancreas, insulin is a very special type of protein made for a very special and specific function critical to diabetes. Working throughout the body, affecting all cell types, insulin's main purpose is to stimulate cells to take up glucose from the bloodstream and transport this glucose into the cell's interior. To do this, cells must have receptors on their surfaces that interact with insulin, creating openings in the cell wall to allow passage of glucose into the cell. Think of a cell as a tiny fortified city on the bank of a busy river and imagine that the supplies for this city are delivered by ships passing through locked gates. In the body, the bloodstream is like the river that carries supplies to the cell wall and it is insulin that serves as the key that unlocks the gate, allowing the supplies, in this case, glucose, to enter the cell once the gate is opened. Diabetes develops when insufficient glucose enters the cell to meet the cell's energy needs and accumulates in the bloodstream. Two conditions must be met to provide adequate glucose for the cell; there must be enough insulin keys to open the gates, and, very importantly, the locks on these gates must work properly. Correspondingly, there are two types of diabetes, type I in which the insulin keys are lacking and type II in which the insulin receptors, or locks, malfunction."[5]

Another aspect of Type 2 diabetes involves the small intestine and what are known as incretin hormones. During a meal, the small intestine absorbs glucose, delivering the glucose to the blood. In response to glucose absorption, two incretin hormones are secreted. The intestine releases glucagon-like peptide GLP-1 and glucose-dependent insulin atrophic polypeptide GIP. They signal increased levels of glucose which then causes the secretion of insulin from the beta cells of the pancreas.[6]

With diabetes, the communication lines between these incretin hormones to the beta cells are impaired. An enzyme DPP-4 gets in the way of the GLP-1, causing releasing of insulin to end too quickly. The GLP-1 also suppresses the release of the hormone glucagon, which releases stored glucose or glycogen in the liver. Also, GLP-1 slows the process of metabolizing food. Since the GLP-1 hormone can become less effective in Type 2 Diabetes, there are now medications that help make the GLP-1 hormone more effective like Trulicity, Victoza, and Bydureon taken by injection. Also Ozempic® (semaglutide) and Mounjaro (tirzepatide) another medication in this category which I explain for weight loss in #11—Eat carbs last as you slowly eat.

> **Watch:** "Trulicity (Dulaglutide). What does it do and how do I use it?" at https://www.youtube.com/watch?v=x_8mfR1Jkes There are also DPP-4 inhibitors like Januvia and Onglyza.

> **Watch:** "DPP-4 Inhibitors in Action" at https://www.youtube.com/watch?v=Ixk_wDPtPfk

So how can we mimic the design of the body? What is the body doing when we eat? Measures glucose amounts. Glucose comes from carbohydrates. So, we should count our carbohydrate intake—count carbs, as well as know what our blood glucose level is. The fewer carbs you eat results in less stimulation of insulin, which causes more fat storage. So it would help to eat fewer carbs per day, under a hundred grams or even less. As a Type 1, I inject insulin. Using short-acting insulin like Humalog and Novolog, I take it about fifteen minutes before eating the calculated number of carbs I plan to eat. I do this if my blood glucose is over 120 mg/dl. If my blood glucose is less than 100, I take the insulin right before my first bite, and if it is 70 mg/dl, I wait about twenty minutes into the meal. Yes, timing is important. *"There is a time for everything, and a season for every activity under the heavens"* (Ecclesiastes 3:1).

#5 Eat breakfast and all meals with fewer carbs and more protein. Eat fewer carbohydrates for every meal. Portion control is the principle.

"Wise People Keep Themselves Under Control: Portion Control, Healthy Choices, and Self-Control"

"If you find honey, eat just enough. If you eat too much of it, you will throw up" (Proverbs 25:16 NIrV). *"It is not good to eat too much honey, nor does it bring you honor to brag about yourself"* (Proverbs 25:27 NCV).

Robert Buynak, M.D., in his book "Dr. Buynak's 1-2-3 Diabetes Diet," gives an accurate formula for determining how many calories to eat each day and maintaining your current weight. The formula is current weight x 11 = daily calories. For example, your weight is 230 pounds x 11 = 2500 calories per day. Since it takes 3500 calories to equal one pound, if you subtract 500 calories per day, you should lose one pound per week. That is, until you reach a plateau of loss. If that happens, you can always try #14 Intermittent Fasting. How many of those calories should be carbohydrates? The Joslin Diabetes Deskbook recommends 40 % of the 2000 calories as carbohydrates, 800 calories (800/4 calories per gram), or 200 grams of carbohydrate per day.

Since carbohydrates directly affect blood glucose levels, the less you eat, the better your blood glucose control will be.

What is the ideal amount of carbohydrates to eat per day? Some advocates of a low-carb meal plan really mean low-carb! Some suggest up to 12 to 15 grams of carbs per meal, comparable to eating just one slice of bread. For the day, they suggest no more than 50 grams. If that is what it takes to keep blood glucose in control, do it! But if you can eat more, maintain blood glucose levels near normal, and lose weight, do it! I usually eat about 15-20 grams for breakfast and 30-35 grams for dinner (lunch) and supper, and an additional 12-15 for snacks during the day (or 90-110 grams per day, which equals 27 % carbs for my weight of 145 lbs.). To determine the grams of carbohydrates in various foods, go to www.calorieking.com. Using the FreeStyle Libre continuous glucose monitoring system, I've been above 140 mg/dl less than 20 % of the time with a 105-110 average.

The carbohydrates to eat should raise blood glucose levels the least. Numbers have been assigned based on research on how fast a particular carbohydrate will make blood glucose rise in two hours compared to an equal quantity of pure glucose. Researchers compared all carbohydrates to glucose, giving the baseline number 100. The smaller the number is, the better the results will be for maintaining good blood glucose levels. The glycemic load (GL) number is for the "typical" serving. The result of each food number they give at www.glycemicindex.com. They put the results into three categories based on the glycemic index number. The following list has the best carbohydrates to eat with the least effect on blood glucose:

Low: 55 and under (<10 GL). Examples include apple, fresh, medium (38 GI, 6 GL, 4 oz, 15 Carb grams), banana, fresh, medium (52 GI, 12 GL, 4 oz, 24 Carb grams), black beans, cooked (30 GI, 7 GL, 4/5 cup, 23 Carb grams), black-eyed peas, canned (42 GI, 7 GL, 2/3 cup, 17 Carb grams), brown rice, cooked (50 GI, 16 GL, 1 cup, 33 Carb grams), carrots, peeled, cooked (49 GI, 2 GL, ½ cup, 5 Carb grams), carrots, raw (47 GI, 3 GL, 1 medium, 6 Carb grams), cherries, fresh (22 GI, 3 GL, 18 cherries, 12 Carb grams), chickpeas or garbanzo beans, canned (42 GI, 9 GL, 2/3 cup, 22 Carb grams), French green beans, cooked (0 GI, 0 GL, ½ cup, 0 Carb grams), grapefruit, fresh, medium (25 GI, 3 GL, 1 half, 11 Carb grams), grapes, green, fresh (46 GI, 8 GL, ¾ cup, 18 Carb grams), green peas (48 GI, 3 GL, 1/3 cup, 7 Carb grams), honey (55 GI, 10 GL, 1 Tbsp, 18 Carb grams), kidney beans, canned (52 GI, 9 GL, 2/3 cup, 17 Carb grams), kidney beans, cooked (23 GI, 6 GL, 2/3 cup, 25 Carb grams), 28, 7), lentils, brown, cooked (29 GI, 5 GL, ¾ cup, 18 Carb grams), lentils, red, cooked, (26 GI, 5 GL, ¾ cup, 18 Carb grams), lima beans, baby, frozen (32 GI, 10 GL, ¾ cup 30 Carb grams), navy beans, canned (38 GI, 12 GL, 5 oz, 31 Carb grams), peach, fresh, large (42 GI, 5 GL, 4 oz, 11 Carb grams), peanuts (14 GI, 1 GL, 1.75 oz, 6 Carb grams), pear halves, canned in natural juice (43 GI, 5 GL, ½ cup, 13 Carb grams), pear, fresh (38 GI, 4 GL, 4 oz, 11 Carb grams), peas, green, frozen, cooked (48 GI, 3 GL, ½ cup, 7 Carb grams), pinto beans, canned (45 GI, 10 GL, 2/3 cup, 22 Carb grams), pinto beans, dried, cooked (39 GI, 10 GL, ¾ cup, 26 Carb grams), rolled oats (42 GI, 9 GL, 1 cup, 21 Carb grams), seeded rye bread (55 GI, 7 GL, 1 oz, 13 Carb grams), sourdough rye (48 GI, 6 GL, 1 oz, 12 Carb grams), sourdough wheat (54 GI, 8 GL, 1 oz, 14 Carb grams), strawberries, fresh (40 GI, 1 GL, 4 oz, 3 Carb grams), sweet corn, whole kernel, canned, diet-pack, drained (46 GI, 13 GL, 1 cup, 28 Carb grams), sweet potato, cooked (44 GI, 11 GL, 5 oz, 25 Carb grams), tomato, chopped (28 GI, 2 GL, 1 cup, 8 Carb grams).[7]

For a good explanation of carbohydrates, watch "How do carbohydrates impact your health?—Richard J. Wood" at https://www.youtube.com/watch?v=wxzc_2c6GMg

By eating fewer carbohydrates per meal, you should eat **more protein**. Half your body weight is the recommended number of grams of protein you should eat daily. The Joslin Diabetes Deskbook lists several benefits of eating more protein, such as a sensation of fullness, maintaining muscle mass while losing weight, better uptake of glucose by muscles, and reducing the spike up of blood glucose after meals.[8] Eat healthy protein. Think of eating fish, turkey, and chicken. We've used many delicious low-carb chicken recipes from Paleo Magazine.

The following from Calorieking.com are the calorie values of one ounce of meat. The amount of protein per ounce is about 7 to 8 grams. Roasted turkey breast, without skin, has 38 calories. Cooked pink salmon has 42 calories. White tuna (Albacore), canned in water and drained, has 36 calories. Rotisserie chicken breast, without skin, with original seasoning, has 42 calories. 96% Fat-free ham, sliced, has 31 calories. Now notice the contrast of highly concentrated saturated fat protein like sausage and ground beef. Fresh beef sausage, cooked, has 94 calories. Ground beef, 95% lean, 5% fat, pan-browned, has 55 calories. Ground beef, 80% lean, 20% fat, pan-browned, has 77 calories. For each ounce of sausage, you can eat three ounces of fat-free ham or turkey breast. It is obvious which one will fill you up. I'm choosing the fat-free ham or turkey breast. What about you?

#6 Focus on staying positive every day with gratitude.

One of the first things to do to start the day is to jot down good things that happened the previous day. (You could do this in the evening before bed as sleep preparation too.) Then give thanks to God for them. Looking at the brighter side of life is the principle.

"Count Your Blessings, and You Will Show a Profit.
Have the Attitude of Gratitude.
Look on the Brighter Side of Life—The Good News."

"Whoever seeks good finds favor, but evil comes to one who searches for it." (Proverbs 11:27).

"A cheerful look brings joy to your heart. And good news gives health to your body" (Proverbs 15:30).

"A cheerful heart makes you healthy. But a broken spirit dries you up" (Proverbs 17:22 NIrV).

"Hearing good news from a land far away is like drinking cold water when you are tired" (Proverbs 25:25 NIrV).

Health benefits from the practice of gratitude have been shown from extensive scientific research by Robert Emmons, Ph.D., when at the University of California at Davis, by researchers at the University of Pittsburgh, University of Manchester, University of Pennsylvania, and the University of Michigan and more. From this research, a practice of gratitude contributes to sleeping better, exercising more, reducing levels of the stress hormone cortisol, feeling more optimistic and connected with others. Also, people who practice gratitude have better compliance or adherence to a meal plan and taking their medications.[9]

Watch: "Robert Emmons: What Good is Gratitude?" at Robert Emmons: What Good Is Gratitude? https://www. youtube.com/watch?v=aRV8AhCntXc

Watch: "Yale's Most Popular Class Is Teaching Students How To Lead Happier Lives | NBC Nightly News" at https:// www.youtube.com/watch?v=tarn7tJk5NE

Here are three ways to practice gratitude. Have you ever had thoughts like these? I have. "It happens over and over. Yesterday, for example, I followed my prescribed meal plan almost perfectly, and I even skipped dinner. So I woke up this morning, and my blood sugar was 300. This is ridiculous. Why should I bother even trying."

It's easy to complain about the bad things happening in our lives, but it takes more effort to think about the good things. When we consider all the things available today to help manage diabetes, compared to how it's been in the past, we can put those things on a "Feel Good Page" and be thankful. Medications like Ozempic, Mounjaro, and Jardiance; new insights into nutrition, fasting, and movement; and new tools like insulin pens, insulin pumps, and glucose monitors you can list on the "Feel Good Page." The way of wisdom teaches us to focus on that page!

"Pleasant words are like honey. They are sweet to the spirit and bring healing to the body." (Proverbs 16:24). *"He who seeks*

good finds goodwill, but evil comes to him who searches for it" (Proverbs 11:27). The first point is to list what is good on your "Feel Good Page." Make sure you list the seemingly insignificant trivial things too. You shouldn't take them for granted. We should look for minor things. Count them. List them. Pray about them. For example, we can have a good day using our **hands** in the yard or garden or at our computer, **see** the beauty of flowers, and enjoy the **aroma** and **taste** of delicious food with gratitude! To see, walk, taste, feel, "eat, as well as have a home," bed, clothes, family, and friends are the little things we should appreciate and not take for granted!

Watch: "After Growing Up Homeless, Boy Is Over The Moon For His New Bed | NBC Nightly News" **https://www. youtube.com/watch?v=vJ0eC88Km-0**

Secondly, talk to yourself in a positive, encouraging, and reaffirming way. Dr. Gary Arsham, a medical doctor with Type 1 Diabetes for more than sixty years, wrote this. "You are the best available source of support for living well with diabetes. You are always there, and you know yourself well; no one else can take care of you as well as you can." Take to heart those words and then add these affirmations from Dr. Richard Beaser of the Joslin Diabetes Center. "I am a strong and self-assured individual, so that when monitoring or scheduling requirements affect my activities with others, I handle my needs without giving in to group pressures. I feel comfortable with and am able to educate those around me about why I need to frequently check and count my carbohydrates. I feel comfortable in my ability to make appropriate adaptations so that I can participate in social activities that I enjoy."

So after listing good things on your "Feel Good Page" and talking to yourself in a positive, affirming way, add this third way to develop more gratitude—comparing yourself to others. Have you ever compared yourself with others? If you were to do so, what would be the best way to do it? Saying, "I wish I were like so-and-so," or saying, "I'm glad I'm not so-and-so." "I wish I was healthier, wealthier, and wiser like so-and-so." If you practice this approach, it can bring envy or resentment instead of gratitude. Better to say, "I'm glad I'm not like so and so." For example, when I was recovering from surgery, I was in a hospital wing for only people with diabetes.

A twenty-seven-year-old blind patient was in the room next to me. He blamed everyone for his situation except himself. Instead of using the click button at his bed to call a nurse, he would rant and rave like a madman. Sometimes he would also bang on the wall while ranting, which was the wall that separated our rooms. He had been in and out of the hospital with diabetic ketoacidosis DKA, which is a condition that results from the lack of insulin for an extended period. This results in a toxic way of metabolizing food for energy, resulting in a concentration of free fatty acids, dehydration, and loss of fluid which brings fewer electrolytes like potassium, chloride, and sodium and an increase in counter-regulatory hormones like glucagon and cortisol. I believe this did not have to happen to him if he had just learned to use the principles we've examined. So this is the comparison: "I'm glad I'm not like this twenty-seven-year-old, being bitter and blaming others for his diabetes self-management."

You could make the same type of comparison with James Havens. Doctors diagnosed James with diabetes in 1914. He became the first American to receive insulin in 1922! To see the whole picture of how few resources were available to live with Type 1 Diabetes, read his story in the second part of this book.

Regarding resource devices, the following is an example of devices that directly relate to diabetes management and should be appreciated. The good news is glucose meters to check what our glucose levels are. For my first twenty-one years with diabetes, glucose meters did not exist! Now with a tiny amount of blood, we can check glucose levels with results in five to six seconds. But it hasn't always been that way! My first glucose meter was an Ames I purchased in the summer of 1981. You had to be near a sink and have a large drop of blood to use it. You then placed the blood on the strip, pushed a button on the meter, and a one-minute countdown would start. Once a minute had elapsed, I would apply a high-pressure dose of water from a small bottle to the strip, washing away what blood had not absorbed into the strip. The strip was then ready to be inserted into the meter for another one-minute countdown. Finally, after following these procedures, which took over two minutes, the result would be displayed. Do you see why the Way of Wisdom principle of good news and gratitude applies to what we have available today? *"A cheerful look brings joy to your heart. And good news gives health to your body"* (Proverbs 15:30 NIrV).

Now more innovative ways to check blood glucose are available—continuous glucose monitoring systems. No finger pricks with a lancet are required. Instead, a painless scan is all that is needed to know what your blood glucose is. For example,

Dexcom, Medtronic, and Abbott offer user-friendly systems. Abbott calls theirs The Freestyle Libre system. It uses a scanning device called a Reader or an app for a smartphone. All you have to do is place it about one inch over a sensor attached to the back of your arm. The Reader then scans from the sensor, which lasts for fourteen days, what your blood glucose level is. The reading is from the interstitial fluid, not directly from the blood. The sensor, about the size of two stacked quarters, is easily attached to the back of your arm. A tiny filament remains just under the skin in the arm's interstitial fluid (We've all heard our bodies are composed of about 55-60 % fluid). Glucose first enters the bloodstream before it seeps into the interstitial fluid. So, there is a short lag between the glucose readings from continuous monitoring systems and a blood glucose meter. Using the trend arrow on the Reader, whether it points up or down, indicates that your blood glucose is currently a little higher or lower than the glucose number shown. I enthusiastically recommend these devices for your use! If you are low or high, the Reader will recommend you do a blood glucose meter check. We can list these devices on our "Feel Good Page." For more information, go to https://freestylelibre.us/

Watch at Youtube: "See More, Manage Better" https://www.youtube.com/watch?v=-q8ixdYZCco&t=47s

#7   **Move Often Throughout the Day: Stand Up, Strengthen Up, and Stretch Out**

"Don't Just Sit There, Keep Moving"

"Go to the ant, you sluggard; consider its ways and be wise! It has no commander, no overseer or ruler, yet it stores its provisions in summer and gathers its food at harvest" (Proverbs 6:6–8). *"From the fruit of their lips people are filled with good things, and the work of their hands brings them reward"* (Proverbs 12:14). *"All hard work pays off. But if all you do is talk, you will be poor"* (Proverbs 14:23 NIrV). *"Ants are creatures of little strength, yet they store up their food in the summer"* (Proverbs 30:25). Remember that when Solomon wrote these proverbs, most work involved manual labor. The principle is to move often throughout the day.

Move often is also good news for blood glucose control. Just getting up out of our chairs and leisurely walking for a couple of minutes every thirty minutes can make the difference. Research indicates that postprandial (after a meal) glucose is lowered from potential highs by half. Not only are glucose high levels reduced, but exercise also lowers cholesterol and triglycerides, and levels of lipoprotein lipase increase. This enzyme aids in the breakdown of fat in the bloodstream.

More good news comes from a study that analyzed the difference a fifteen-minute leisure walk after a meal would make on blood glucose levels compared to just sitting. Picture your blood glucose as a daunting ice-capped mountain peak by sitting compared to an image of safe, green rolling hills by walking. By just sitting, you will see your blood sugars climb higher and higher to the peak, but walking can cut the rise in half. So, I've learned to take a short walk after a meal rather than sit.

And here is an additional benefit. Walking reduces insulin levels and makes your muscles more sensitive to insulin. It takes tremendous exercise to burn seventy calories, the amount in a slice of bread. So, that is not why exercise benefits better health; instead, it cuts back on insulin resistance. When you take a walk for a few minutes, your body becomes more sensitive to insulin for the time you are walking and up to the following 48 hours. How long can you breathe before becoming fatigued? Have you ever thought about that? As you read this, you are still breathing. You aren't exhausted, and that is because of the abundance of mitochondria in the muscle cells. They are tiny energy producers. The muscles with the most mitochondria, like the heart, have a slow contraction speed and slow twitch conduction, not fast like your hand muscles have. You can exhaust your hand muscles by using them too much. Your breathing muscles' activity is aerobic because the mitochondria aid the cells as tiny energy producers, providing oxygen and fatigue resistance. So, when we start walking, the leg muscles do not fatigue because they are abundant with mitochondria. When you walk, there is a response for less insulin needed, which can last for up to 48 hours. Insulin resistance reverses, and blood sugar comes down.[10]

When I walk, I speed up my pace and even jog for half a block. This is called **interval training** or intermittently speeding up the pace. People with Type 2 Diabetes who usually walked 10,000 steps daily participated in a twelve-week study of picking up the pace for part of their daily steps. They walked their typical 10,000 steps but increased their speed for part of their walks. As a result, they experienced an increase in how well their insulin worked—insulin sensitivity. Dr. Colberg, an exercise expert with Type 1 Diabetes, mentions several good benefits of this exercise, such as burning more fat and glucose, improving blood glucose control, strengthening the heart, and extending the calorie-burning power of muscles after workouts.[11]

For a good formula to determine intensity using your heart rate, look at the article "Exercise Intensity: How to Measure It" by the Mayo Clinic.[12]

Watch: "Have Type 2 Diabetes? Try Walking After Eating" at https://www.youtube.com/watch?v=itmdsOUVBcc

Watch: "Walk for Health: The Best Medicine" at https://www.youtube.com/watch?v=mbIM1LTfytQ

Stand Up

Books have been written with titles like "Sitting Kills, Moving Heals: How Everyday Movement Will Prevent Pain, Illness, and Early Death—and Exercise Alone Won't" by Joan Vernikos, Ph.D. or "Get Up!: Why Your Chair is Killing You and What You Can Do About It" by James Levine, MD. Dr. Vernikos was the Director of NASA's Life Sciences from 1993 to 2000, while Dr. Levine has worked for the Mayo Clinic. From the research discussed by both authors, too much sitting can harm health. If we spend up to an hour exercising per day, what do we do the other twenty-three hours? Dr. Joan Vernikos recommends using gravity to our advantage. By just slowly standing up, valuable changes occur in our body—like muscle contractions and nerve stimulations. One benefit of doing this is better blood pressure levels. The process of standing up is the stimulus, not the amount of time standing. The way to get the most benefit from standing up is to do it slowly and to stand up at least thirty-two times a day. "Stand up, sit less, move more" summarizes research on avoiding sitting too much.

Standing has its own benefits. For example, Dr. Francisco Lopez-Jimenez's editorial on a research study of "Replacing sitting time with standing or stepping" summarizes the benefits of standing and stepping instead of sitting. The benefits are improved fasting blood glucose and triglyceride levels, and a prevention of atherogenesis (formation of abnormal fatty or lipid masses in arterial walls). Also, standing up and adding some steps will improve weight control.[13] If you work at a desk, research indicates a 20-8-2 ratio for every thirty minutes—sit for twenty minutes, stand for eight, and move for two.[14]

Dr. Joan Vernikos also gives this example of how beneficial standing up can be. Her 99-year-old uncle was hit by a car as he crossed the street. His upper leg bone, the femur, was broken. He was hospitalized. As he was lying in his hospital bed, he called her, asking her what to do. She told him to get out of the hospital as soon as possible, but in the meantime, to sit up every 30 minutes with his legs hanging over the side of the bed, after doing this a couple of minutes to lie back down. Once he was home, she advised him to stand up every 30 minutes. He followed her prescription when he got home, and to the amazement of the orthopedic surgeon, his bone healed in two weeks. So, let's stand up slowly more than thirty-two times daily for health and vitalization.

Strengthen Up

One of the most important factors to know about strength training is the benefits this exercise brings for blood sugar control. The reason is that muscle contractions uptake glucose into the cells of the muscle through another avenue without the use of insulin. Your muscles can continue to bring in more glucose via Glut4 glucose transporters — without insulin initially — for some time after exercise. The muscle stores glucose or glycogen and uses it as an energy source during exercise. When dieting, many people lose not only fat but muscle, too. Think of the muscle as your gas tank or glucose tank that replenishes the expended glycogen supply by uptaking glucose from the blood during and after exercise without insulin and with insulin too. So, it makes your insulin much more effective and sensitive, with less of it needed. In other words, by maintaining muscle mass or increasing the amount of muscle, the body becomes more sensitive to insulin. So, strengthen and build up your muscle mass for better blood sugar control.

When is the best time to do this type of exercise? By doing this after meals, I've discovered I can maintain better blood glucose levels. I am up to eight exercises three times a week with four sets of repetitions for each exercise. I do several exercises for about fifteen minutes after two meals a day. I rotate the exercises of the upper body and lower body muscles every other day. A proper sequence of breathing is essential, too. Breathe out while actually lifting the weight and breathe in while lowering the weight. Don't hold your breath when lifting the weight because high blood pressure can result!

Stretch Out

After you do your strength training exercises, follow them with **stretching exercises** while the muscles are warm, says exercise expert Dr. Sheri Colberg. Some of the benefits she lists are moving and reaching more fully and relaxing stiff, sore, and tired muscles. Also, lowering the risk of sports injuries, preventing falls due to lack of flexibility, and combating the loss of flexibility from aging, inactivity, and diabetes are additional benefits.[15]

Motivation to Exercise

It is amazing what we can do when we have the motivation and see the benefits. Here is an example of someone who overcame insurmountable obstacles and succeeded in training for an Ironman competition. Picture yourself running a 26.2-mile marathon, riding a bicycle 112 miles, and swimming 2.4 miles. Winners in Ironman Triathlon races accomplish all of this in less than fourteen hours. Endurance is needed. No one would doubt Ironman competition is very difficult. It is named "Ironman" not because competitors wear iron suits but because the event is hard, like iron. Ironman Triathlons require willpower. Without training, competing in this competition would be dangerous and ill-advised. We can imagine riding a bicycle around a few blocks in our neighborhood, but who could pedal 112 miles altogether?

This competition is for the young, although there is an instance of 85-year-old Hiromu Inada participating in the race and completing it in 16 hours and 53 minutes. Average winning times are 12 hours and 35 minutes. The willpower of some people is incredible, which brings me to the example of 39-year-old Jay. Not only did he train and compete in this event, but he did so while battling brain cancer. He first saw an Ironman race on TV in 1989 and thought, "they must be superhuman." When his daughter was born, he wanted to show her that she could do unbelievable things, and he would compete when she turned ten. But he started his training early when his daughter was only three. On that day in 2018, when he was diagnosed with brain cancer, he started his training. Last year his finishing time was 13 hours and 40 minutes. This accomplishment came after two brain surgeries, 30 radiation sessions, and a year of chemo.

His performance did not just happen; he had great motivation. During 2020, because of COVID-19, athletes could make their virtual courses. Jay set his finish line in front of his house. When he came around the corner, straining toward the finish line, he could see his home with his wife and daughter (and hundreds of others) cheering him toward the tape. He said, "My daughter and my wife were holding that tape, so I just zeroed in on them, thinking, 'I'm coming home.' I didn't have much energy, but I kissed my wife and got down on my knees to say to my daughter and hero, 'If I can do it, you can do it. Dream big and never give up hope.'" In this scene, we see the motivation that gave him willpower—his family. When it comes to exercising in Wise Way #7, let's focus on the benefits exercise brings for our health and wellness and be motivated by our families, friends, and potential friends we can encourage to practice them![16]

Read this article, "Get Stronger, Live Longer," for descriptions of eight exercises and images of how they are done with neoprene dumbbells.

https://assets.aarp.org/www.aarpmagazine.org_/articles/ health/fitness_machines/SmartFitness_FreeWeights.pdf

Stretching exercises are illustrated in this pdf.

"Exercises for Older People." https://www.nhs.uk/Tools/ Documents/NHS_ExercisesForOlderPeople.pdf Inserted

11.8.19— https://www.nhs.uk/livewell/fitness/documents/ NHS_sitting_exercise.pdf

For a full explanation of the benefits of exercise, read the article "The Science of Exercise" in Diabetes Forecast magazine. http://www.diabetesforecast.org/2010/jul/the-science-of-exercise.html

CHAPTER TWO

Wise Ways to Stay in Control During the Afternoon

"She (wisdom) will give you a garland to grace
your head and present you with a glorious crown.
Listen, my son, accept what I say, and the years
of your life will be many." (Proverbs 4:9-10).

#8   Stay Hydrated

Drink Cold Water—
*"Like cold water to a weary soul is good news
from a distant land"* (Proverbs 25:25).

Remember, when reading the proverb above, the statement
made of God's wisdom teachings in Proverbs 4:22—*"They are
life to those who find them and health to one's whole body."* The
basic meaning of the word *proverb* is to represent, compare, or
be like. Proverbs are pictures of reality. What better way to picture the gratifying, exuberant effect that good news has on a
person than with the image of the satisfaction cold water gives a
thirsty person? *"Like cold water to a weary soul is good news from
a distant land"* (Proverbs 25:25).

Proverbs have more than one dimension, and the meaning here is not just about good news. In other words, the consequence of good news is pictured with the wonderful feeling that cold water gives to a thirsty person. And guess what? Cold water is good for our health.

I recently visited a worker at a supermarket. I overheard her tell a customer how she was feeling with her diabetes. Then, I had a short visit with her. She told me that she drinks water to bring down her blood glucose level, which amazingly works sometimes. Why? Dehydration makes a person feel fatigued. It can also elevate the stress hormone cortisol. Cortisol is a counterregulatory hormone to insulin. Thus, when cortisol levels are elevated, insulin is less effective. The result is elevated blood sugar levels.

Drink Water! *"Like a snow-cooled drink at harvest time is a trustworthy messenger to the one who sends him; he refreshes the spirit of his master."* (Proverbs 25:13). Doctor Willett of Harvard Medical School teaches drinking sixty-four ounces of water a day for a person on a 2,000-calorie meal plan.[17] Others have suggested drinking half an ounce for every pound you weigh and an ounce for every minute you exercise to keep hydrated. French researchers discovered drinking thirty-four ounces of water per day prevented elevated blood glucose in a nine-year study of 3600 individuals.[18] Eating whole foods rich in water also makes a difference in the amount to drink. Most fruits and vegetables are mainly water. Notice the water content in the following foods: fruits and vegetables (80–95%), hot cereal (85%), low-fat fruit-flavored yogurt (75%), boiled egg (75%), and fish and seafood (60–85%). When we compare a popular junk food like potato chips, we discover it has only 2 percent water content.[19] What about carbonated soft drinks? According to Doctor Willett, these drinks work for staying hydrated but are loaded with sugar. And sugar-free artificially sweetened soda drinks are a concern. Many are wary of artificial sweeteners.[20] If that is a concern, get an Infuser for fruit-infused water!

A way to determine dehydration is the color of urine. For example, the dark yellow or yellowish-brown color could indicate dehydration.[21] "Studies have shown that being just half a liter dehydrated can increase your cortisol levels," says Amanda Carlson, RD, director of performance nutrition at Athletes' Performance—a training clinic for world-class athletes. "Cortisol is one of those stress hormones. Staying in a good hydrated status can keep your stress levels down. When you don't give your body the fluids it needs, you're putting stress on it, and it's going to respond to that," says Amanda Carlson.[22] Dehydration can elevate blood glucose because cortisol levels can increase, causing resistance to insulin. In addition, with fewer bodily fluids, blood decreases, also causing low blood pressure.

Another consideration for weight loss is to drink water. Are you hungry or just need to drink something? Feeling hungry may signal the need for more fluids. How can you distinguish thirst from hunger? Sip a glass of ice water before grabbing something to eat, and then wait five to ten minutes. Thirty-six ounces of cold water daily can elevate metabolism and calorie burning by one hundred calories per day, a study reveals. A benefit of drinking water cold comes when drinking ice cold water. Ice cold water requires energy to warm it to core body temperature.[23]

How many calories will you burn to bring an ice-cold

sixteen-ounce drink to body temperature? One calorie is burned for each ounce of iced beverage to warm it to core body temperature. Drinking sixty-four ounces of ice-cold water a day results in burning sixty-four calories.[24] Staying hydrated and drinking ice-cold water is vital for those with health concerns, which is all of us, isn't it? Wisdom's way teaches, *"The mind of a person with understanding gets knowledge; the wise person listens to learn more"* (Proverbs 18:15 NCV).

I drink small amounts of water throughout the day—six glasses with six to eight ounces of water each time. To drink it all at once isn't good for you! I combine drinking water with eating water-rich foods like vegetables and fruit. *"The wisdom of the prudent is to give thought to their ways"* (Proverbs 14:8).

#9   Wisely Eat Healthy Snacks

Does An Apple a Day Keep the Doctor Away?

"Make plans by seeking advice; if you wage war, obtain guidance" (Proverbs 20:18). We all like snacks, but some snacks are unhealthy, like donut holes. So, to win the war against poor health, we need guidance or advice to make wise choices for snacks. If you follow an intermittent fasting schedule, like 16 hours of fasting and an eight-hour window for eating or 18:6, time will be the first factor for restricting snacks. No snacks that will break your fast! You can drink black coffee, tea, or water and non-calorie flavoring. I will recommend intermittent fasting in the 14th wise way. Knowledge is knowing a tomato or avocado is a fruit; wisdom is not putting it on a fruit salad. Knowledge is knowing donuts, donut holes, chips, pretzels, and a bucket of

buttered popcorn at the theater are snacks; wisdom is replacing them with healthy snacks! What are the benefits of snacking? Snacking helps prevent overeating at meals, and it provides a constant source of nutritional fuel. The body also gets a regular supply of fuel, which can help prevent low blood glucose levels when using insulin or sulfonylureas like Glipizide, Glimepiride, and Glyburide. Of course, before fasting, consult your doctor if you are on medications like these.

What are some good snacks to eat? I would cautiously eat fresh fruits in small quantities because they stimulate insulin production. So when eating an apple, it should be a small portion like half or a cup or four ounces of cherries, half of a grapefruit, twelve or fewer grapes, and half of an orange, peach, or pear. These are good snacks from the criteria of being low-glycemic. A popular snack is a donut hole, or should we say donut holes! A single donut hole weighs only half an ounce and has fifty-two calories! Whereas 5.1 ounces of strawberries have only forty-six calories! Which one will give you a more-full feeling for a snack? Low-calorie density foods, which add more volume of food to your snack, are also high-density nutrient snacks. One donut hole has sugar, saturated fat, and flour. In contrast, the 5.1-ounce serving of strawberries has virtually no fat but has water and three grams of fiber. When we subtract the fiber, it has only thirty-four calories and anti-inflammatory antioxidants (antioxidants stop or delay damage to the cells). Strawberries have omega 3 and 6 fatty acids, minerals like magnesium, potassium, and calcium, and vitamins like A, C, E, and K. So eat low–glycemic index carbohydrates that don't spike up blood sugars.

Raw vegetables are even better snacks. Eat them with a lower-fat dip or with different flavored mustards. At our Diabetes Support Group, one person told me she's enjoying eating radishes and losing weight. Radishes? Yes, she's eating radishes. Radishes are rich in fiber, vitamin C, and potassium. One cup of raw radishes has only 19 calories and 4 grams of carbohydrates, but 1.7 grams of fiber. Another person said he's been eating mushrooms and has noticed better blood glucose control. Mushrooms have 23 calories for one cup with 2 grams of carbohydrates. They are also anti-inflammatory foods.

Radishes and mushrooms are much better choices than potato chips and pretzels. They are more filling. Radishes are about 90% water. In comparison, potato chips have about 2% water. One serving (28 grams) of chips has 160 calories, 15 grams of carbohydrates, and 10 grams of fat. One serving (28 grams) of pretzels has 100 calories and 23 grams of carbohydrates. Do not eat these for snacks!

Deli meat wrapped in romaine lettuce leaves, low-fat cottage cheese and fruit, a boiled egg, smoked salmon, or tuna with vegetables would all be good options. Remember, the calories add up quickly in nuts like almonds, walnuts, and pecans. Portion control is essential for nuts! Again, the calories add up quickly.

What about eggs? Here are what two individuals say about the benefits of eating eggs—Dr. Jason Fung and Dr. Eric Berg. First, notice what Dr. Fung writes. "Potential egg nutritional benefits include increased weight loss, better skin and eye health, enhanced liver and brain function and a reduced risk of heart disease and metabolic syndrome. Free-range eggs, in particular, tend to be safer, more ethically produced and higher in several important nutrients. Studies now conclude that eating eggs, even daily, does not raise the risk of heart disease. In fact, consuming lots of eggs reduces the risk of diabetes by 42 percent."[25]

Dr. Eric Berg says this in a Youtube presentation. "Egg protein has the greatest anabolic effect—48% of egg protein is converted into body protein. This means it goes directly into your muscles and joints. Your body is only able to convert 32% of the protein in meat and fish." Studies have shown that if you consume whole eggs, your body is more efficient at building muscle and you have a shorter recovery time after exercise. The insulin index is a scale that classifies how different non-carbohydrate foods affect insulin. Whole eggs have a much lower effect on insulin than egg whites alone. When you remove the fat from a protein source, you have a greater insulin spike." Dr Berg eats 4 eggs per day. I eat an average of three eggs per day. Do your research and make a wise decision.

Dr. Josh Axe, DNM, DC, CNS, is a certified doctor of natural medicine, doctor of chiropractic, and clinical nutritionist. He lists on his website "51 Healthy Snack Ideas." His ideas with recipes include such snacks as "Baked Cinnamon Apple Chips, Five-Minute Healthy Strawberry Yogurt, Paleo Apple 'Nachos,' Raw Homemade Applesauce, Very Cherry Snack Bar, Cajun Roasted Chickpeas, Zucchini Chips, Crispy Chickpea Bites, Healthy Spicy Black Bean Dip, Healthy Sweet Potato Nachos, Paprika and Chili Kale Chips, Quick Crackers, Creamy Avocado Yogurt Dip, Spiced Nuts, Roasted Pumpkin Seeds, Spicy Buffalo Cauliflower Bites and many more. Go to https://draxe.com/healthy-snack-ideas/ to read the recipes.

Watch: "Travel Foods & Snacks" at https://www.youtube.
com/watch?v=FOeWaR7gJY4&t=10s

#10 Eat Dinner (lunch), Walk, and Take a POWER NAP.

A good conscience is a soft pillow.
I'm so good at sleeping I can do it with my eyes closed.

Why take a nap? Please give me one good reason. Jesus did!
Remember what happened on the Sea of Galilee? *"A furious
squall came up, and the waves broke over the boat, so that it was
nearly swamped. Jesus was in the stern, **sleeping on a cushion"***
(Mark 4:37-38). When was Jesus sleeping? During a storm, yes,
during a storm! We find a wisdom insight on how he could do
this in Proverbs 3. *"**Do not let wisdom and understanding out
of your sight**...Then you will go on your way in safety, and your foot
will not stumble. When you lie down, you will not be afraid; when
you lie down, **your sleep will be sweet"** (Proverbs 3:22-24).

Taking naps has been the habit of many famous people like
Albert Einstein and Winston Churchill. Albert Einstein took
naps! Your IQ may not be off the charts, but when it comes to
naps, you and I can be a genius. Einstein believed in power naps.
He would sit in his chair and hold a pencil or a spoon as he dozed
off. When he dropped it, he knew his nap time was over. Unlike
many daytime nappers, Einstein also got plenty of rest at night,
regularly sleeping for at least 10 hours. Winston Churchill said,
"Nature has not intended mankind to work from eight in the
morning until midnight without that refreshment of blessed
oblivion which, even if it only lasts twenty minutes, is sufficient

to renew all the vital forces... Don't think you will be doing less work because you sleep during the day. That's a foolish notion held by people who have no imaginations. You will be able to accomplish more. You get two days in one — well, at least one and a half." We could add more than Nature, but wisdom, God's wisdom, would condone taking a nap, as seen in Jesus! Dr. Sara Mednick, in her book "Take a Nap; Change Your Life," gives 20 reasons why we should take a nap. Some of the reasons relate to diabetes self-management. The Ninth reason she gives is that sleepy people are more susceptible to junk food cravings. The eleventh reason is to reduce your risk of diabetes or better manage it. Studies reveal sleep deprivation increases cortisol levels. Cortisol, the stress hormone, causes a need for more insulin. Increased levels of cortisol bring resistance to insulin, which then has a direct effect on blood glucose management.[26]

Dr. Mednick reports that sleeplessness causes hypertension, but during sleep, blood pressure decreases. So, when you remain awake longer than normal, your blood pressure can stay higher. This can also result in a higher risk for strokes. In addition, when we deprive ourselves of sleep, we enter a period of overdrive and need extra energy to support physical functions. Also, irritability, anger, depression, and mental exhaustion can be linked with sleeplessness. Dr. Mednick gives these guidelines for napping: keep the room as dark as possible, go for quietness, and stay warm.

"I usually take a two-hour nap from one to four," said Yogi Berra. What is the optimal length of time for a nap? Various lengths of a nap bring different beneficial results. If you have time to nap as long as Yogi, you will sleep through all the stages

of sleep. If you don't have that kind of time, even a twenty-minute nap brings benefits. Those twenty minutes help with rejuvenated alertness and improve motor skills like typing. Thirty to sixty-minute naps or slow-wave sleep brings better decision-making and short-term memory but grogginess when waking. So, during a twenty-minute power nap in the lighter stages of sleep, increased energy and alertness come when awakening. Avoid taking caffeine for up to four hours before you expect to take your nap, and then your nap will become your energy drink!

According to a recent study, one way to remedy the negative effects of a poor night's sleep is to take a short nap the following day.[27] Researchers have found naps to reduce stress and bolster the immune system. The Mayo Clinic lists the following benefits of taking naps: relaxation, reduced fatigue, increased alertness, improved mood and performance, including quicker reaction time and better memory.[28] So, take a nap as your energy drink!

#11 Eat Carbs Last as You Slowly Eat.

Precious Present

"It is not good to have zeal without knowledge, nor to be hasty and miss the way" (Proverbs 19:2). Someone says, "I've always enjoyed my food. I may eat fast, but it's often because...Well, actually, I've never thought about why I eat fast, but it doesn't really matter, does it?" "Whoever is patient has great understanding" (Proverbs 14:29). The following is an example of how patiently eating brings about great understanding for wise mindful eating.

How do we eat? The table is set and ready for food. Twelve hungry brothers sit at the table ready to eat. Mom brings the food and sets it before them. The food is limited and these guys are famished. Can you picture the scene? The only thing you hear is the chomping of teeth. How long will it take for them to clean their plates? I can imagine asking for dessert in five minutes. When you sit down to eat you're not sitting with eleven hungry brothers are you? Yet, it is so easy to fall into the trap of devouring food without even tasting it.

Imagine a tiger chasing you. Running for your life a sharp deep cliff confronts you. You have no place to go. The tiger is getting so close you can feel him breathing down your neck, then you notice a rope dangling over the cliff and grab it. Holding onto the rope for your life, you sway, dangling from the cliff. The tiger roars above and five hundred feet below sharp jagged rocks invite you to fall. Then you notice two mice chewing on the rope above you. What should you do?

The tiger above, the rocks below and the rope is about to break! Just then you notice delicious-looking bright red, ripe strawberries growing out of the side of the cliff. You stretch out one hand, pluck a strawberry, and pop it into your mouth. The strawberry is so sweet and refreshing. You think "Delicious— that's the best strawberry I've ever tasted."

If you were still occupied with the tiger above or the sharp rocks below, you would have never tasted and enjoyed the strawberries. We call this the *precious present*! When we eat, are we focusing on the smell, texture, color, and rich taste of the food we're eating? Research indicates for most people, the feeling of satiety (fullness) takes about twenty minutes. We haven't given ourselves time for that feeling to catch up because we're gulping down our food!

Sleep Deprivation

Physical health is also impacted by sleep deprivation. There is an impairment of hormones that relate to appetite. Less leptin, the "feel full" hormone is released, and more of ghrelin, the "still hungry" hormone. This makes losing weight an even greater challenge. So, the strategy is to sleep more and lose weight. Adequate sleep relates to the feeling of satiety and to this strategy of eating slowly. Synergy is needed when these two principles of sleep and satiety come together and give you greater results than expected.

Eating Sequence: Eat Carbs Last

So, what can we do? Previous studies have found that eating quickly results in eating more! Eating too fast outpaces the satiety signal (feeling full sensation), which takes about 20 minutes. Could "postprandial" (after meal) blood sugar levels be affected by how fast you eat carbs? Yes, especially if you eat the carbs on your plate first. What is the timing sequence of eating protein and carbs? Eat protein first! What difference does that make? "You've got to be kidding?" God's wisdom instructs us to be mindful of sequence. For example, *"Finish your outdoor work and get your fields ready; after that, build your house"* Proverbs 24:27. "Carbohydrates raise blood sugar, but if you tell someone not to eat them — or to cut back drastically — it's hard for them to comply," says Dr. Louis Aronne. Researchers at Cornell say, "This study points to an easier way that patients might lower their blood sugar and insulin levels." The research focused on how much and when carbohydrates are eaten. Eleven Type 2 Diabetics who were obese and only on metformin were the research group. Their meals consisted of carbohydrates, protein, vegetables, and fat. They ate carbs first and then waited fifteen minutes to eat protein. Then, they reversed the order. Their blood sugars were checked post-meal every 30, 60, and 120-minute intervals. Eating carbs last brought much better results with 30, 60, and 120-minute checks — by about 29 percent, 37 percent, and 17 percent, respectively.

The Importance of Eating Fiber

A curious factor is shown when we look at food labels. Under the total number of carbohydrates listed, fiber is included. Fiber is a carbohydrate that the body cannot break down, and it has several benefits. Eating foods with fiber means you eat fewer calories, which is also helpful for controlling weight. The book "Glucose Revolution" lists these three superpowers of fiber: First, it reduces the action of an enzyme that breaks starch down into glucose molecules. Second, it slows down stomach emptying: when fiber is present, food moves more slowly. Finally, it creates a dense mesh in the small intestine, making it harder for glucose to reach the bloodstream. Through these designs, fiber slows down the breakdown and absorption of any glucose that lands in the stomach after it. This results in flattening the spike up of glucose. And let me add that this is especially true of soluble fiber, which dissolves in water, becomes a gummy gel, and helps blunt elevated blood glucose after a meal. So fiber (soluble) limits rapid BG peaks, gives a full feeling longer, and helps control cholesterol. A man's goal is to eat 30 grams of fiber per day, and a woman should eat 20 grams per day.

Another way of putting these benefits from the book Glucose

Revolution is this. "Fiber is also good for our glucose levels for several reasons, notably because it creates a dense mesh in our intestine. The mesh slows down and reduces the absorption of molecules from food across the intestinal lining. What does this mean for our glucose curves? First, that we absorb fewer calories. And second, with fiber in our system, any absorption of glucose or fructose molecules is lessened."[29]

"Better to have a dish of vegetables where there is love than juicy steaks where there is hate" Proverbs 15:17. Most people find a delicious steak meal satisfying to the taste, but the taste is lost when eating the meal with bitter, resentful, and hateful people toward you. Whereas eating a meal with those you love is pictured with vegetables. And guess what? As we've been examining, vegetables are good for us. Isn't it interesting that a subtle message of a meal of vegetables shows love? And what are vegetables? They are very beneficial for health. Here are some examples of fruits and vegetables rich in soluble fiber. Start your meals with greens. Any vegetable qualifies, from roasted asparagus to coleslaw to grilled zucchini and grated carrots. We're talking artichokes, broccoli, turnips, brussels sprouts, eggplant, lettuce, tomatoes, and also beans.

Broccoli

Dr. Josh Axe website says this about broccoli. "Broccoli was first cultivated as an edible crop in the northern Mediterranean region starting in about the sixth century B.C. As far back as the Roman Empire, it's been considered a uniquely valuable food when it comes to promoting health and longevity. Believe it or not, it didn't actually become widely known in the U.S. until the 1920s, which is surprising if you consider how popular it is today. Why is broccoli good for dieters? It's one of the most nutrient-dense foods on Earth. One cup of the cooked veggie has just over 50 calories but a good dose of fiber (2.3 grams), protein and detoxifying phytochemicals (which reduce inflammation). Is broccoli a carb? As a complex carbohydrate high in fiber, it is a great choice for supporting balanced blood sugar levels, ongoing energy and helping you feel full. Want to know a secret to losing weight fast? Including more high-volume, low-calorie, high-nutrient foods in your meals is key. Broccoli nutrition is high in volume due to having a high water content, so it takes up room in your stomach and squashes cravings or overeating without adding lots of calories to meals."[30]

Soluble Fiber

Here is a contrast between high soluble fiber raw vegetables like bell peppers and carrots which have very little impact on blood sugar levels compared to dry cereal like Rice Krispies. I did a check on my blood sugar and discovered that just twenty-three grams of Rice Krispies with four grams of milk almost doubled my blood sugar level from 100 mg/dl to 175 mg/dl in less than forty minutes.

In contrast to dry cereal, beans are loaded with fiber and especially soluble fiber. The following list gives serving size, total fiber grams per serving, and the number of soluble fiber grams in each serving. Black beans ½ cup 6.1, 2.4 Kidney beans, light red ½ cup 7.9, 2.0 Lima beans ½ cup 4.3, 1.1 Navy beans ½ cup 6.5, 2.2 Pinto beans ½ cup 6.1, 1.4. The best options to keep your glucose levels steady are berries—Strawberries 1 ¼ cup 2.8

(1.1), citrus fruits—oranges 1 small 2.9 (1.8), and apples—with skin 1 small 2.8 (1.0) because they contain the most fiber and the smallest amount of sugar. The worst options—because they have the highest amount of sugar—are mangoes, pineapple, and other tropical fruit. Make sure you eat something else before you eat the fruit. Eat fruit last. It makes a good dessert.

Eating Whole Foods

Eating healthy is a challenge, especially when there are so many delicious unhealthy temptations. People think that if they practice some portion control, they will succeed. Like Yogi Berra said, "When the waitress asked if I wanted my pizza cut into four or eight slices, I said, 'Four. I don't think I can eat eight." People use fad diets to shed pounds quickly. But, unfortunately, once the weight is lost, the old habits return, and so do the pounds and then some. Dr. Jennifer Hubert of St. Joseph Health Medical Group calls this yo-yo dieting. Dr. Hubert says, "Other findings indicate that yo-yo dieting may lead to a higher risk of increased body fat, which means these diets, in the long run, can have the opposite of the intended effect of losing weight. What's worse is that most yo-yo dieting is done with the trendy diets of the moment, which are poor nutritionally compared to eating a regular diet of whole foods like this video is showing."[31]

Whole foods are like the difference between an apple and apple juice. The way to have fruit is in its whole state, with all the nutrients still there. Plus, in the whole state, foods are much more filling! Healthy whole foods are naturally loaded with fiber, vitamins, and minerals. Some are antioxidants that protect cells against damage. Whole foods are rich, nutrient-dense foods. They have no added sugars and fats and exclude added salt or other high-sodium ingredients.

Three More Ways to Disarm the Effects of Carbs on Blood Glucose

When my wife and I were on a trip recently, we went to eat at a restaurant. Before leaving my hotel room, I ate some nuts. Once there, I ordered some thick bacon, scrambled eggs with a variety bowl of fruits, and a biscuit. Once the waitress brought the food, I ate my bacon and eggs first and then cut my biscuit in half and ate it with some of the fruit. After eating, I took a fifteen-minute walk back to the hotel. My blood sugar stayed within 100 to 140 mg/dl.

Why am I telling you this? Since carbohydrates directly affect blood glucose levels, use fat to blunt or disarm their effects. Fifteen minutes before you eat your meal, eat some cheese and nuts. And here is why? Fat will affect the pyloric sphincter, a valve from the stomach to the small intestine. The fat causes it to begin to tighten, which causes the absorption of carbohydrates to slow and helps prevent a glucose spike. The pyloric valve is a muscular ring that regulates the speed by which food leaves the stomach and goes into the intestine.

Dr. Rob Thompson writes, "As soon as fat passes through your pyloric valve and reaches your intestine, it activates a reflex that closes the pyloric valve, which keeps food from exiting the stomach. It doesn't take much fat to do this. Scientists have found that as little as two teaspoons (10 g) of fat before a meal will slow stomach emptying. If you eat a fatty snack— a piece of cheese or a handful of nuts— 10 or 15 minutes before a meal, it will close the pyloric valve. When you sit down to eat, you will still have plenty of room in your stomach to enjoy your meal. However, because the tightened pyloric valve slows the passage of food out of your stomach, it takes less food to fill you up. You'll ultimately end up eating less."[32] So eat some cheese and nuts fifteen minutes before a meal for this to happen.

Another thing I did on this trip at another meal was to eat a bowl of salad with vinaigrette dressing first. I've discovered an effortless thing you can do is eat or drink vinegar. Why? Because it slows down the process of breaking down the complex carbohydrates into glucose. The enzyme that does this is amylase. Dr Rob Thompson writes this. "Vinegar inhibits amylase and has been proven to slow the absorption of starch in humans. It has been used for centuries to treat Diabetes. Studies show that 2 tablespoons (30 ml) consumed before eating starch lowers the after-meal glucose and reduces demands for insulin. Vinegar doesn't have to be consumed straight. It can be sprinkled on food as a condiment— a common practice in Mediterranean countries— or used in a salad dressing."[33]

The third thing I did on my trip to disarm the glucose spike effect of carbohydrates was walk after eating, not nap. Do that after you walk. The time of walking is essential. When you walk for a few minutes, your body becomes more sensitive to insulin for the time you are walking and up to the following 48 hours. Plus, your body uses two avenues to reduce blood glucose levels after eating. Insulin is one avenue, and the glucose tranporter— Glut4. As I mentioned in #7, research indicates you can potentially reduce by half how high your blood glucose will elevate. So do these three things to help control blood glucose: eat cheese and nuts fifteen minutes before eating, eat a salad with some vinegar dressing, and take a short walk after eating.

Walk With the Wise Like Thomas Edison

If you can't seem to eliminate junk food, then don't give up. Instead, look to those who didn't give up even under very trying situations, like Thomas Edison! Edison described himself as deaf, but in fact, he was not totally deaf. It is more accurate to say he was very hard of hearing. He once wrote, "I have not heard a bird sing since I was twelve years old." So, why didn't Edison invent a hearing aid? He often told reporters that he was working on one; sometimes, he tested hearing aids designed by others. But it seems that Edison saw advantages to being deaf. For example, he said that it helped him concentrate on his work. In 1927, he told a group of 300 hard-of-hearing adults, "Deaf people [like himself] should take to reading. It beats the babble of ordinary conversation." Thomas Edison's labs burned in 1914. He said, "Our greatest weakness lies in giving up. The most certain way to succeed is always to try just one more time." The way of wisdom states that *"A wise man has great power and a man of knowledge increases strength"* (Proverbs 24:5). The best way to do "one more time" is with more knowledge.

105-Year-Old Ida Keeling

The following story tells of a woman winning a race at one hundred-five years old. When I read her story, I was impressed with her insights about living. Ida Keeling won and broke the world record for her age group—100 years old at the 122nd Penn Relays. Ida didn't start running until she was sixty-seven! A family tragedy of the murder of her two sons motivated her daughter, Shelly Keeling, to enroll her in a 5K run. "She was just sitting at home in gloom. I just picked her up one morning and said, 'You're coming with me,' and I bought her an extra pair of sneakers, and the rest is history." What is her secret to longevity? "Eat for nutrition, not for taste," she said. "Do what you need to do, not what you want to do, and make sure you exercise at least once every day." And as an afterthought in the story, She said, "I thank God every day for my blessings." And why not![34]

Guidelines Summary of Eating Slowly and Eating Carbs Last

The Joslin Diabetes Center has a program called "Why WAIT? Weight Achievement and Intensive Treatment for Diabetes." Mindful eating is taught.[35] Take your time. Don't get in a big hurry in eating. They suggest relaxing and taking a couple of minutes of deep breathing. Look at the food, noticing its color and texture. (Pretend you will get a grade on a 200-word description you will write of the food!) Smell the food, inhaling the aroma before taking your first bite. Serve yourself less food than you think you need. Taste and savor every bite, chewing it thoroughly. To slow down your pace of eating, put down your fork between each bite. Before deciding to go back for seconds, wait twenty minutes.

And follow these ideas. Take a sip of water between bites. If eating with others, pace yourself with the slow eater. Avoid the "just one more helping" request. Leave some food on your plate. Pre-regulate consumption by deciding how much to eat prior to the meal.

Watch: "Why WAIT? Weight Achievement and Intensive Treatment for Diabetes" at https://www.youtube.com/ watch?v=9r_Aw70TZGE

Watch: "Love to Eat? How to Eat and NOT Gain Weight" https://www.youtube.com/watch?v=cF_zd1LxkuE

CHAPTER THREE

Six Wise Ways in the Evening

"I instruct you in the way of wisdom and lead you
along straight paths. When you walk, your steps
will not be hampered; when you run, you will not
stumble. Hold on to instruction, do not let it go;
guard it well, for it is your life" (Proverbs 4:11-13).

#12 Use Tools Throughout the Day—
Fitness Trackers, etc.

Yogi Berra on travel gear: "Why buy good
luggage, you only use it when you travel."

For the best blood glucose management results, use tools. Proverbs 14:4 states, *"Where there are no oxen, the feed box is empty. But a strong ox brings in a great harvest."* In ancient times, oxen were essential farming equipment (compare Deuteronomy 22:1, 10). Remember these proverbs are *"life to those who find them and health to one's whole body"* (Proverbs 4:22). The application is not oxen for our health, but tools like food scales, measuring cups, food labels, smaller plates, walking shoes that give comfort and support, a clock for timing of meds, meals, and pedometers or fitness trackers for movement, record booklets or health apps and glucose meters or continuous glucose monitor systems like the FreeStyle Libre, Medtronic Guardian 4, or Dexcom g7. So, good tools will equip us for better health.

One of the best tools for counting carbs in whole foods is the EatSmart™ Digital Nutrition Scale, which calculates carbs, fiber, and fats. There is a database with nutritional values for a thousand foods. For example, the number of apples is 002. After removing the core and placing the apple on the scale, the scale will show the total calories with grams of carbohydrates and fiber.

Watch: EatSmart™ Digital Nutrition Scale "Weight Loss Tool—Count Calories—EatSmart Nutrition Scale" at https://www.youtube.com/watch?v=AbM4Fbf9OPU

A pedometer or fitness tracker is one of the best motivational tools for getting more steps each day. Researchers conducted a study with two groups wearing pedometers. The participants in one group wore a pedometer with a goal of 10,000 steps daily. The other group's goal was to take a brisk, thirty-minute walk daily. The pedometers worn by the brisk, thirty-minute-a-day walking group were non-viewable. The group using the viewable pedometers averaged over 10,000 steps per day. In comparison, the thirty-minute walking group only walked an average of 8,270 steps—a difference of almost a mile per day.

The following are comments from participants in the 2001 Diabetes in Control 10,000-step research study on the benefits of using a pedometer: "I reduced my stress levels." "It was very easy to just put on the pedometer and check it during the day—it really works." "I never thought I could get to ten thousand steps a day, but just by tracking my steps and increasing ten percent a week, I was able to do it!" "I was surprised to see that it became a habit after just a short time." "My whole family wanted pedometers, and they also increased their steps." "Just by removing the remote controllers, we picked up four hundred steps." "My dog is healthier than ever (I wore the pedometer, not the dog)." "I have more energy, and my blood sugars have never been better. Now my doctor is wearing a pedometer." "My blood pressure is down to normal." "My clothes all fit better." The following are more beneficial tools to use.

Plate Size: "Brian Wansink, Mindless Eating"
Interview concerning plate size and how the size helps with portion control at **https://www.youtube.com/watch?v=mP5AFkWZ3eY**

How much movie theater popcorn do people eat? Does it depend on how hungry they are or how good it tastes? Could the size of the box influence how much one eats? Dr. Wansink did a study to determine the influence of the box size on the amount eaten. At a theater in Chicago at a 1:05 p.m. showing, people were given a free box of popcorn. Researchers gave some of them a large box and others a medium-sized box.

They asked participants to answer a few concession stand questions after the movie. They were also to return their bucket or box with any uneaten popcorn. The only catch was they didn't tell the participants the popcorn was five days old. They did keep it in sterile conditions. Participants were told, "We have found that the average person who is given a large-size container eats more than if they are given a medium-size container. Do you think you ate more because you had the large size?" Most of the participants disagreed. They thought the container size did not affect the amount one would eat. The big-bucket group ate 173 more calories than the medium-sized group. They ate 53 percent more than those with medium-sized boxes. The conclusion was that people eat more when given a bigger container!

What would be a good application for using that information on a daily basis? For example, if you spoon four ounces of sweet potatoes onto a twelve-inch plate, it will look much less than if you had spooned it onto an eight-inch plate. Why not put your food on a midsize plate instead of a larger plate, giving it the appearance of holding more food? We all need to restrict the amount of food we eat to the proper portion size. This could be an easy strategy to use to aid with that goal. The way of wisdom says, *"The wise in heart are called discerning"* (Proverbs 16:21).

Calorie-free salad dressings: Walden Farms no calorie dressings—https://www.waldenfarms.com/

Shoes: Go-Walk Skechers Shoes

Pedometers and Fitness Trackers: (They monitor different actions like tracking daily steps and measuring heart rate and sleep quality. My family uses the Fitbit Charge 2, 5, or Inspire.)

Introducing Fitbit Charge 5 In-Depth Review https://www.youtube.com/watch?v=c7KHBR-xSlc

Labels: "Label Reading 101" at https://www.youtube.com/watch?v=MrdCBqFYDyo

Always when looking at labels, count the carbs. Since the body does not metabolize the fiber, subtract the amount. Doing this is very important for those with ratios to determine how much insulin to give to cover the carbs eaten. The greater the saturated fat, the longer the body metabolizes the carbohydrates. If you use an insulin pump, use the dual mode to extend the amount of time the insulin is delivered. When you see sugar alcohol on the label, you should calculate half the amount for insulin ratios because half is metabolized and affects blood glucose levels.

If you were instructed to keep good records of your blood sugar readings, the amount of food you eat each day, and the number of steps you take each day, would you say, "You've got to be kidding"? Or "I've never done such a silly thing"? However, the way of wisdom states the concept with this principle: *"Be sure you know the condition of your flocks"* (Proverbs 27:23). Most of us do not have flocks, but we each have a body, and we need to keep track of a herd of health issues like the condition of our blood glucose levels, blood pressure, amount and quality of sleep, exercise and movement and foods. In other words, we need to keep a daily personal health inventory. One way to do this is to keep a food diary along with records of blood glucose readings. Mynetdiary or Fitbit Charge are two of many apps available. Using a tool like this helps with weight loss. In the *Journal of the American Dietetic Association*, an article titled "Food Records: A Predictor and Modifier of Weight Change in a Long-Term Weight Loss Program" concluded: "Those who most accurately recorded their food consumption lost the most weight."

Mynetdiary App. Watch: "MyNetDiary Overview" https://www.youtube.com/watch?v=gVAjjkPsAY4

Ozempic and Mounjaro

Research studies prove Ozempic (semaglutide) causes weight loss. One study showed that participants in a trial lost 10-15% of their body weight over a little more than a year with weekly Ozempic injections combined with healthy eating and exercise. Only 2% of people in the placebo group lost weight, but in the Ozempic group, about 75% lost 5% or more of their body weight. There is another innovative medication called Mounjaro, whose result for weight loss for 84 weeks was 26.6%.

Ozempic and Mounjaro are new medications that have brought outstanding results for people with Type 2 diabetes, including losing weight. We have two people in our diabetes support group taking Ozempic. They take a once-a-week injection and do much better with blood sugar control. They also have suppressed hunger, resulting in tremendous weight loss. What do these medications do? They increase insulin sensitivity while inhibiting the liver from releasing glucagon to help lower blood sugar levels. They also suppress appetite and slow digestion, causing many people to lose weight. Due to its long duration of action, people take it once weekly, making it convenient.

They are two among many GLP-1 agonists. They increase the effectiveness of this incretin hormone messenger for insulin production. After you eat, cells in your intestines release GLP-1. They trigger insulin release and block glucose release from the liver. They also slow down how fast food leaves your stomach, making you feel full. GLP-1 is also thought to directly affect the appetite control area of your brain, as well as certain hunger hormones.[36] The GLP-1 can act on brain neuronal circuits in the hypothalamus involved in appetite control. The difference between the medications is that Mounjaro (tirzepatide) is a dual GLP-1/GIP receptor agonist. This means it increases the activity of gut peptides that promote satiety, while GIP also stimulates lipolysis—the breakdown of fat for energy use. Dr. Beverly Tchang says, "We think tirzepatide's weight loss effect is driven more by the GIP component than the GLP-1 effects, and this may be the reason why we are seeing more weight loss from tirzepatide than with other medications, which are only GLP-1 agonists."[37]

#13 Eat supper (dinner) earlier with less saturated fat and carbs.

"Eat Breakfast Like a King, Lunch Like a Prince, and Dinner Like a Pauper"

Wisdom's way teaches the following on the importance of timing:

"Anyone who refuses to work doesn't plow in the right season. When he looks for a crop at harvest time, he doesn't find it" (Proverbs 20:4 NIrV).

"Finish your outdoor work. Get your fields ready. After that, build your house" (Proverbs 24:27).

"A person finds joy in giving an apt reply— and how good is a timely word!" (Proverbs 15:23).

"It is not good to have zeal without knowledge, nor to be hasty and miss the way" (Proverbs 19:2).

Researchers in Spain studied 420 participants in a 20-week weight-loss treatment program.[38] The research answered, "Could the timing of when you eat, be just as important as what you eat?" The meal with the most calories was the lunch meal. They ate forty percent of their daily calories at lunch. The timing of when to eat was the factor analyzed to determine if the time made a difference in weight loss. Researchers divided participants into two groups—early eaters and late eaters. The early eaters ate their lunch before 3 p.m., and the late eaters any time after 3 p.m.

Those who lost significantly less weight and at a slower rate were in the late eaters group. In that group, they ate fewer calories for breakfast and often skipped breakfast. Insulin resistance also increased. But instead, eat breakfast like a king, but be sure to cut back on carbohydrates. Ideally, eating fifteen grams of carbohydrates along with plenty of eggs will help you maintain better blood glucose levels. "Our results indicate that late eaters displayed a slower weight-loss rate and lost significantly less weight than early eaters, suggesting that the timing of large meals could be an important factor in a weight loss program," said Frank Scheer, Ph.D., assistant professor of medicine at Harvard Medical School, and senior author on this study. Not only will eating late make it easier to gain weight, but it also makes it more challenging to maintain blood sugar control. So, the lesson is to try to eat the evening meal early. The amounts of fat and carbohydrates will also determine your blood glucose management.

Someone says, "Your blood glucose is affected by sugar and carbs, so avoid them. Don't worry about other types of food!" However, wisdom's way says, *"The mind of a person with understanding gets knowledge; the wise person listens to learn more"*

(Proverbs 18:15 NCV). Is fatty food just the shy, harmless guy sitting in the back row? When you eat fatty foods, they have a powerful metabolic punch. Free fatty acids (FFAs) in the blood increase with high–saturated fat meals. What does that do? Insulin resistance increases with high–saturated fat meals with carbohydrates. With that resistance, you need more insulin to break through the insulin resistance barrier. This compounds blood glucose control for those with Type 1 diabetes and many with Type 2 diabetes with high insulin resistance.

Eating saturated fat like in a hamburger also changes the timing of the rise in blood glucose after a meal. Fat takes up to six hours to move through the gastrointestinal tract. Whereas rapid-acting insulin such as Novolog, Humalog, or Apidra and the new Fiasp (I highly recommend because it becomes active in two minutes instead of 15 to 20 like the others) stay active for just four hours. When you eat a high-fat meal, a significant amount of glucose remains after the four-hour life of the rapid-acting insulin. This results in elevated blood glucose readings. For example, Red Robin's Bacon Cheeseburger has 71 grams of total fat, with 24 being saturated. The burger also has 50 grams of carbohydrates. One effective way to combat this is to get your hamburger lettuce wrapped instead with a bun, leaving off the cheese and carbohydrate bun.

The following are the American Heart Association's guidelines for fat consumption: Limit total fat intake to less than 25–35 percent of your total calories daily and limit saturated fat intake to less than 7 percent. This means a 2000-calorie meal plan could include 140 calories from saturated fat, or 16 grams. It is also best not to eat those 16 grams in one sitting.

Reduce consumption of saturated fats like red meat and dairy products. Think chicken, turkey, and almond milk. Monounsaturated fats like olives, avocados, cashews, almonds, peanuts, and olive and peanut oil lower LDL ("bad") cholesterol and insulin resistance and raise HDL. Polyunsaturated fats are found in salmon, herring, tuna, cod, pumpkin, sunflower seeds and oil, and corn oil. They also lower LDL cholesterol and triglyceride levels. Instead of using canola oil which is highly processed, use coconut oil, olive oil, and organic butter. Dr. Axe says, "Despite unjustified warnings about saturated fat from well-meaning, albeit misinformed, experts, the list of butter's benefits is impressive: Butter is full of vitamins, minerals, and MCFA that greatly benefit overall health." However, the amount used in one sitting matters for blood sugar control with carbohydrate consumption.

Avoid meals containing 40 or more grams of fat, especially if the fat is saturated. Alter the amount and timing of your insulin if you eat a high-fat meal, taking an additional smaller dose later, especially if you've eaten some carbohydrates with the meal. For people with Type 2 diabetes, taking oral medications and those on insulin, doing some physical activity—for example, walking after a high-fat meal—can help control blood glucose. And by all means, lower the amount of carbohydrates you eat—15 grams or at most 30 grams per meal. And ideally, with a high-fat meal, avoid carbs altogether.

In summary, these are the steps to take for the key to victory. Avoid meals containing 40 or more grams of fat, especially if the fat is saturated. Please keep it to 16 grams a day or 5 per meal. If you decide to eat pizza, eat the thin-crust kind. One piece has 202 calories, 18 grams of carbohydrates, and 4.3 grams of fat. If you eat a hamburger, eat a lettuce-wrapped one and avoid the carbohydrates altogether. And get some exercise after you eat. Research indicates if people sit after a meal, their blood sugar peaks like a mountain for about two hours. The mountains become safe, gentle rolling hills if people take a 15-minute walk at one mph after a meal. With a one mph walk after a meal, you restrict the blood sugar peaks to half the size. So, if your blood glucose is 100, it will increase by 50 points.

When you eat, eat the vegetables first, then the protein, and finally the carbohydrates. Jessie Inchauspe writes, "The slower the trickling of glucose into our bloodstream, the flatter our glucose curves and the better we feel. We can eat exactly the same thing—but by eating carbs last, we make a big difference in our physical and mental well-being. What's more, when we eat foods in the right order, our pancreas produces less insulin. And as I explained in Part 2, less insulin helps us return to fat-burning mode more quickly, the positive results of which are many—and include losing weight."

For a good explanation of fat watch: What is fat?—George Zaidan" at https://www.youtube.com/watch?v=QhUrc4BnPgg&t=7s

#14 Fast—Use time-restricted eating in the evening and morning.

"Man eats too much. Thus he lives on only a quarter of what he consumes. The doctors, however, live on the remaining three quarters." —Ancient Egyptian Doctor

---

"There are multitudes of diseases which have their origin in fullness, and might have their end in fasting."—James Morrison.

The study in #13, about 420 participants—early and late eaters—also relates to this wise way. The largest meal, with 40 percent of daily calories, was eaten before 3 p.m. or after. The early eaters benefitted most from weight loss and blood glucose control.

Another study called "Early Time-Restricted Eating" at the University of Alabama correlates with early and late eaters' research.[39] They studied overweight people on two different eating schedules. One was eating from 8 am to 8 pm and the other only from 8 am to 2 pm. They discovered that more fat was burned by eating during a smaller window of time, the second category. Their research indicates more fat was burned during the night with fewer food cravings during the day. I've used this idea to eat my last meal earlier in the day and especially to not eat after the last meal! I maintain better blood glucose control when I can follow this schedule. (I'm not always able to do so because my blood sugar levels get too low before bedtime. I can't go to bed with an 80 mg/dl, especially when I know the level will drop.) Do your own research. Try avoiding snacks during the evening and before bed. See if your blood glucose improves.

After trying Time-Restricted Eating in the evenings, you could restrict your eating all morning. In other words, do some fasting until noon or one. Then you would have a window to eat for the next six hours. I've done this successfully for better blood sugar control and weight loss. There are several things to consider when trying an 18:6 or 16:8 (fasting for 16 to 18 hours and having an eating window from six to eight hours) fasting schedule. Sixteen hours may seem long, but if you're getting adequate sleep, you should be asleep for about seven hours. These characteristics, like knowledge, self-control, perseverance, and hope, will apply to fasting.

Let's consider the first one on knowledge. *"Wise people have success by means of great power. Those who have knowledge gather strength"* (Proverbs 24:5 NIRV). Continuing to fast after an evening of Time-Restricted Eating is an easy way to start to fast because you already have a night's head start. During the morning, have no calories that could stimulate insulin and eat food for energy production. When we eat, our energy source comes from carbohydrates, which the body converts into glucose. Any glucose we don't utilize for energy the body converts into glycogen stored in the liver. And if we overeat and our glycogen stores are full, the carbs are converted to fat. How many times a week should you fast for sixteen to eighteen hours? Since I have Type 1 Diabetes, it depends on how I do in the evening. If I've calculated the grams of carbohydrates and the insulin I take and my blood glucose keeps from getting low, I can fast. I watch my blood glucose with my continuous glucose monitor and lower my basal dose.

However, if you have type 1 diabetes, it is important to remember that ketone levels may rise when you are not eating. This may be a challenge if you need more basal insulin and depend on meal-time insulin to avoid high levels of ketones. The good news is that you can measure your ketone levels. It is also essential to monitor blood glucose levels—hypoglycemia is a risk of fasting.

Benjamin Horne, M.D. gives this caution for those with Type

2 Diabetes on medications. "If you are taking medications that are aimed at reducing the amount of glucose in your blood, together with fasting these can cause potentially fatal hypoglycemia," Horne says. "It's not a minor safety risk." So, consult your healthcare team before trying this if you are on medications to control your blood glucose levels.

The second point is it takes self-control during the morning hours to fast. *"Like a city whose walls are broken through is a person who lacks self-control"* (Proverbs 25:28). City walls were defense mechanisms for ancient cities to defend themselves and keep enemies out. Since many people have breakfast during the morning, how can they manage the hunger pains? By drinking water and other no-calorie beverages, like plain coffee or tea. You will be surprised at how you can ward off hunger pangs.

Another thing we need to do during those morning hours is not succumb to temptations. Keep snack food out of reach and out of sight. By doing this, you can persevere and reap great rewards for your health. *"Let us not become weary in doing good, for at the proper time we will reap a harvest if we do not give up"* (Galatians 6:9). What is happening with your body as you fast? It helps to know so that you can endure and not give up. Here is a basic outline of what I've read happens. For the first eight hours, blood sugars fall, food has left the stomach, and the body produces minimal insulin for basal metabolisms like breathing and the heart. Does your BMR stop working during sickness? The basal metabolic rate, or BMR is the amount of energy required to support the work of the heart, brain, lungs, and other organs at rest, in the absence of any physical or mental exertion, says Boris Draznin, M.D. Then, for the next four hours, the digestive system sleeps, the body begins healing, and human growth hormone increases. During hours twelve through eighteen, this is what happens.

Food consumed has been burned, the digestive system goes to sleep, the body begins the healing process, human growth hormone begins to increase, and glucagon is relaxed to balance blood sugars during the twelve and thirteenth hours. After fourteen hours, the body has converted to using stored fat as energy, and human growth hormone starts to increase dramatically.[40]

Here are six benefits of having increased growth hormone: Increased muscle strength, better fracture healing, enhanced weight loss, stronger bones, reduced heart disease risk, and better mood and sleep. After fourteen hours of fasting, the body begins to use stored fat as energy, and after sixteen hours, it begins to ramp up the fat burning.

To lose weight, have you ever experienced your body having a plateau effect? You get to a certain weight loss, and then you can't seem to lose another pound? This is where fasting is so beneficial. Instead of your fat-burning rate slowing down to conserve energy, it ramps up. One research study showed an increase of 12%.

Following an intermittent fasting diet can make maintaining the weight you lost over the long term easier. A two-part study of 40 obese adults, published in Frontiers in Physiology in 2016, compared the combined effects of a high-protein, low-kilojoule (foods such as fruits, vegetables, and legumes are less energy-dense foods), intermittent-fasting diet plan with a traditional heart-healthy diet plan. The results showed that while both diets proved to be equally successful in reductions in body mass index (BMI) and blood lipids (fatty acids and cholesterol), those on the intermittent-fasting diet showed an advantage in minimizing weight regain after one year.

So here is another benefit called hope, not wishful thinking. *"Hope deferred makes the heart sick, but a longing fulfilled is a tree of life"* (Proverbs 13:12). One person in our diabetes meetings uses intermittent fasting daily and needs a new wardrobe because of weight loss. I call that hope, not just wishful thinking. Fasting works for a healthier life!

#15 Have a good night's sleep.

> *"My son, do not let wisdom and understanding out*
> *of your sight...When you lie down, you will not be*
> *afraid; when you lie down, your sleep will be sweet...*
> *When you walk, they will guide you; when you sleep,*
> *they will watch over you; when you awake, they*
> *will speak to you. (Proverbs 3:21, 24; 6:22).*

Some people claim they can get by with just four or five hours of sleep per night. How many hours of sleep are needed? The Centers for Disease Control recommends, along with the Mayo Clinic, no less than seven hours a night. Many people aren't getting enough sleep. One in three adults reports they sleep an average of six or fewer hours a night.[41] The millions of people using Fitbit health-trackers only get six-hours and thirty-eight minutes per night.[42] Drowsy driving is an ever-present dangerous result of sleep deprivation. According to the Centers for Disease Control, an estimated one in twenty-five adult drivers reports falling asleep while driving in the previous 30 days. Drowsy driving is also estimated to cause 72,000 crashes, 44,000

injuries, and 800 deaths in 2013. These numbers are underestimated, and up to 6,000 fatal crashes each year may be caused by
drowsy drivers.[43]

Physical health is also impacted by sleep deprivation. There
is an impairment of hormones that relate to appetite. Less
leptin, the "feel full" hormone is released, and more of ghrelin, the "still hungry" hormone. This makes losing weight an
even greater challenge. So, the strategy is to sleep more and
lose weight.[44] Studies also reveal that cortisol levels increase
the next evening after just one night of sleep loss, causing insulin resistance. Also, the efficiency of the immune response is
damaged as well as an increase in inflammation with lack of
sleep.[45] A lack of sleep also lowers the levels of the chemical
serotonin, which then results in pain sensitivity increasing as
well as increased feelings of anxiety. To compensate for lower
levels, the body compensates with cravings for carbohydrates.[46]

When we sleep we are not just dreaming and wasting time.
Our bodies are designed to use that time to stay or get healthy!
Several processes are happening as we sleep. According to the
National Sleep Foundation, such health benefits as "muscle
repair, memory consolidation and release of hormones regulat-
ing growth and appetite" are happening. This prepares us to
concentrate and make decisions for all day time activities. As we
sleep, we go through several stages of sleep. These stages repeat
throughout the night in about ninety-minute cycles. Our bodies are as the psalmist writes, *"Fearfully and wonderfully made"*
(Psalm 139:14).

Fitbit health trackers have divided sleep into three stages—
light, deep and REM sleep. Imagine a maintenance crew working

during the light stage. During light sleep, body maintenance is at work keeping a perfect balance, a homeostasis of all bodily functions and hormones. Light sleep is important because it comprises about 50% of sleep each night. With the lack of sleep, several hormones that affect weight will not be in balance such as leptin, ghrelin, cortisol, and growth hormone.[47]

During normal sleep, the metabolic rate is reduced by about 15%. The amount of energy (calories) the body burns to maintain itself is metabolism. That is why my basal rate of insulin in my insulin pump is so low compared to other times of the day—.30 units per hour compared to .90 at breakfast time. I don't need as much energy to supply my needs thus less insulin is needed during the night.[48]

Picture a person's tense arm muscles holding up a shield to deflect incoming harmful arrows. During deep sleep, the immune system is strengthened. Growth hormone is secreted which results in cellular rebuilding and repair. This is also the time the body uses for muscle development.

Also, picture a profile of a person's brain with colorful lights going off within the brain. Processing and storing information happens during the REM (rapid eye movement) stage of sleep. Vivid dreams occur, the body is relaxed and the volunteer skeletal muscles are turned off. Maybe that prevents acting out those vivid dreams. If deep sleep is about the body, REM sleep is about the brain. Mental restoration is taking place so that you can clearly think and decide during the day.[49]

How do you wake up after a night's sleep? Are you groggy and feel like you haven't slept or do you wake up refreshed? I've found my Fitbit Health tracker very beneficial for keeping me aware of the kind of sleep I'm getting. It also identifies how much of the night I'm awake too. This helps me plan my schedule for when to go to bed and when to get up so I can get an adequate amount of sleep. *"The plans of the diligent lead to profit* (health) *as surely as haste leads to poverty"* (Proverbs 21:5).

Certain foods help promote sleep. The Institute of Health Sciences recommends foods that contain tryptophan, which helps induce the production of serotonin, which is required to make melatonin.[50] Melatonin is a hormone that regulates sleep-wake cycles. The body produces more during darkness, preparing the body for sleep. Light has the reverse effect.[51]

Foods that help with this are grass-fed dairy products, nuts, fish, chicken, turkey, sprouted grains, beans and brown rice, eggs, sesame seeds, and sunflower seeds. Eat melatonin-rich foods like bananas, Morello cherries, ginger, barley, tomatoes, and radishes. Include them in your dinner or supper. For a complete discussion on getting to sleep, go to Dr. Josh Axe's (a certified doctor of natural medicine) article "Top 20 Ways to Fall Asleep Fast!"[52]

Difficulty Falling to Sleep?

Why? Jesus himself took naps. Remember what happened on the Sea of Galilee? *"A furious squall came up, and the waves broke over the boat, so that it was nearly swamped. Jesus was in the stern, sleeping on a cushion"* (Mark 4:37-38). What is amazing about this event is that Jesus was sleeping during a storm. Have you ever had difficulty falling asleep? All of us have, but Jesus could sleep even during a storm. How?

God's wisdom gives us a key. *"Do not let wisdom and*

understanding out of your sight...Then you will go on your way in safety, and your foot will not stumble. When you lie down, you will not be afraid; when you lie down, your sleep will be sweet" (Proverbs 3:22-24). *"When you walk, they will guide you; when you sleep, they will watch over you; when you awake, they will speak to you"* (Proverbs 6:22).

Have you ever had a root canal done? The procedure can be excruciating. How do you handle the pain? Meditation helps. I've gone over and over in my mind calming words like *"God is my shield and refuge"* from Proverbs 30:5. *"Every word of God is flawless; he is a shield to those who take refuge in him."* Positive wise thinking can bring a calming effect to a stressful situation. *"Be careful what you think, because your thoughts run your life"* (Proverbs 4:23 NCV). By doing this we keep in our sight wisdom and understanding, which we read brings sweet sleep. *"Whoever seeks good finds favor, but evil comes to one who searches for it"* (Proverbs 11:27). By seeking what is good, listing the good, meditating on the good are all practices of keeping wisdom in sight. These are all methods for having sweet sleep. And we are talking about Jesus' wisdom.

What can easily happen instead of focusing on the good is to focus on problems or worries. Thinking about them over and over again is not conducive to falling asleep. In fact, by meditating on them they are compounded and become independent of reality. These worries can easily become worse and more powerful than they are. This all leads to restlessness and mounting obstacles and hazards for falling asleep. Dwelling on what is good will fight off the anxiety of worry. *"A cheerful look brings joy to your heart. And good news gives health to your body"* (Proverbs 15:30 NIrV).

A ten-week research study with hundreds of participants was done by Professor Robert Emmons, Ph.D., while he taught at the University of California at Davis to demonstrate what effects gratitude might have on health and well-being. They were randomly divided into three groups. One group was a gratitude condition group, and the members were to list five things for which they could be thankful that had affected their lives from the previous week. Another group was the hassle group, and those people were to list five burdens that affected their lives the previous week. The third group was the neutral group, and its members were to list five things, either positive or negative, that had affected their lives the previous week.

The results were then analyzed with several tests. The final analysis was that the people in the gratitude group felt better about their lives, were more optimistic, and exercised more than those in the other groups. The results were even better when gratitude was practiced daily, looking at a variety of blessings.[53]

Several other studies have been conducted with similar results. For example, another ten-week study was done by the Department of Physical Medicine and Rehabilitation at the University of Cal-Davis, involving people with post-polio syndrome. The results of the gratitude group were that the people felt better about themselves, felt more optimistic about the coming week, and felt more connected with others than the other groups. Another significant finding was that they went to sleep quicker, spent more time sleeping, and felt more refreshed in the morning.[54] The idea is that if you want to sleep more soundly, count your blessings, not sheep.

#16 Correct low-blood glucose: hypoglycemia.

Outsmart Hypoglycemia—Eat Smarties

According to Proverbs 24:14, people have hope when they find wisdom, which inspires them not to give up. *"Wisdom is sweet to your soul. If you find it, there is a future hope for you, and your hope will not be cut off."* God's wisdom applies in the following way—to give thought to managing diabetes. *"The wisdom of the prudent is to give thought to their ways...The prudent see danger and take refuge"* (Proverbs 14:8, 22:3).

One of the dangers of diabetes is hypoglycemia. In the "Diabetes Attitudes, Wishes and Needs" research study, researchers found a deep fear of hypoglycemia (blood glucose levels below 70 mg/dl).[55] These episodes can happen at any time during the day. So, being prudent and alert is essential. Hypoglycemia is an acute stress factor for people using insulin or Sulfonylurea medications like Glipizide or Glyburide. Blood glucose can get low when too much insulin is in circulation. Epinephrine (adrenaline) is the "fight or flight" hormone that alerts the body to danger or stressful situations. It produces symptoms of low blood glucose like weakness, hunger, sweating, trembling, "butterflies," and heart palpitations. Epinephrine activates Glucagon. Glucagon releases stored glucose or glycogen in the liver, raising blood glucose levels (glycogenolysis). A person without diabetes might experience some of these symptoms if they haven't eaten for several hours. What I just described are the usual responses for people without diabetes. Still, the normal responses are compromised for those with Type 1 Diabetes or Type 2 on insulin or medications like Glipizide because too much insulin may be in circulation. So, taking carbohydrates to raise the blood sugar level is essential to prevent dangerous lows.

The epinephrine response gets blunted for many people with Type 1 diabetes for a long time. They lose the early warning signs of low blood glucose. Lower and lower blood glucose levels have to occur before their response occurs. So, instead of being in the 60's mg/dl blood glucose levels, it may be less than 40 mg/dl. According to the Joslin Diabetes Center, new research indicates that avoiding hypoglycemia episodes can restore the proper, timely response of the epinephrine, giving the warning signs at a much higher, safer blood glucose level.[56]

A great precaution is to check our blood glucose more often. When not using my continuous glucose monitoring system, I check myself up to twelve times daily. Regularly checking yourself is essential, especially if you are on insulin or the medications previously mentioned. This reduces the risk of having a severe episode! Another precaution is always having glucose tablets, Smarties™, or SweeTarts™ with you. For a visual episode of not taking this precaution while on a walk, watch "Jim's 1st Person Low" at https://www.youtube.com/watch?v=f7SEaZSWqXs

How many grams of quick-energy carbohydrates are needed to treat low blood glucose readings? A good rule of thumb is that 1 gram of glucose raises the blood sugar by 3, 4, or 5 points for body weights of 200, 150, or 100 pounds, respectively. For example, 5 grams of dextrose, as found in Smarties™ or SweeTarts™, raises the blood sugar by about 20 points for a 150-lb person.[57]

Treat a low with 15 grams of Smarties™ or similar candy, then wait twenty minutes and check again. Also, combine a low glycemic index carbohydrate with a fast-acting carbohydrate. For example, I woke up one night at about 2 am to visit the restroom. I checked my blood glucose and discovered it was 46 mg/dl. So, I took 9 grams of Smarties™ (GI of 96) and a small amount of milk (6 grams of carb—GI of 34). When I checked my blood glucose at 6 am, I was 116. Since I weigh about 150 lbs. the 15 grams of carbs should have elevated my blood glucose by 60 points. That number and the combination of carbs increased my blood glucose level by 70 points. Measuring the amount of carbohydrates will prevent overcompensating and ending up with high blood glucose!

As a preventive for hypoglycemia at night, check your blood glucose right before bed. If you take insulin, always know how much insulin is active (Humalog and NovoLog last for four hours). This plan has worked for me in the almost sixty-three years I've had diabetes, preventing ambulance calls and hospitalization (only once in 1991).

#17 Take advantage of opportunities to help others.

To Be Encouraged, Encourage

"A good person gives life to others; the wise person teaches others how to live" (Proverbs 11:30 NCV).

Glenn lived by himself (He had LADA diabetes for twenty years—Latent Autoimmune Diabetes in Adults, a progressively slow-developing Type 1 with his beta-producing insulin cells being destroyed). He picked up a business card at the local pharmacy for the diabetes support group. He started attending the meetings. He encouraged and received support from others who were also facing many of the same challenges with diabetes.

"*A generous person will prosper; whoever refreshes others will be refreshed*" (Proverbs 11:25). He put this wisdom into practice. He became very involved with the community diabetes support group. When several of us would meet to count advertising flyers for a diabetes seminar to mail, he would be there! He knew people would attend because they received one of the mailed flyers. And they would be helped to control their diabetes. He would set up chairs in the large community room at the library for seminar participants. He was helping, being encouraged, and encouraging!

Blood glucose control was a perpetual struggle for him. God has marvellously designed the human body. When we eat carbohydrates, they reach the small intestine, a hormone (GLP1), a messenger, goes to the pancreas and signals for an initial release of stored insulin and manufacturing more. The amount is exact to meet the needs of the number of carbohydrates eaten and will keep the blood glucose in a tight range between 70 to 140 mg/dl. But people like Glenn do not have the beta cells that produce insulin. His body has destroyed them. He required a strict balancing act, which is a great challenge! Someone said that managing diabetes is like playing the piano with your right hand while juggling with your left hand, all while trying to keep your balance as you walk on a tightrope. Managing diabetes is a balancing act!

All Glenn had to do was take his insulin at the right time, in just the right amount, several times each day; check his blood sugars multiple times a day to make sure he wasn't too high or too low; balance the right amount of food with the insulin he took. Stay alert for stress or colds that elevate the stress hormone cortisol causing elevated blood sugars. And also realize he must do this every day because there is never a vacation from diabetes. That's how simple it can be! Ha! People like Glenn need encouragement! We all need to give help and receive help!

There is nothing like experiencing a low, low blood sugar. An extremely low reading is like squeezing out every ounce or milligram of glucose to stay conscious. I've experienced this nightmare situation several times but have stayed conscious. Glenn's blood glucose was a rollercoaster of ups and downs. I called him one afternoon, asking how he was doing. He was out of blood glucose checking strips. He had been having lows, and some were extremely low. I told him my wife, and I would bring him some strips. We found him on his bedroom floor, helpless, sitting with his legs crossed in briefs. His eyes were glazed. He barely recognized me.

Immediately I checked his blood glucose. It was about 20 mg/dl. This was a severe hypoglycemic episode. The race was on to keep him conscious. Since he was awake and could swallow, I gave him Smarties™ from my glucose-checking kit. The Smartiestm eventually brought him out of the severe low. Ten days later, he suffered another severe episode. No one was there to help, and he passed away. Many people need a helping hand. Many have helped me—my wife, parents, friends, doctors, and nurses. One morning I woke up with stickiness on the back of my head—honey. I was so distressingly in a severe hypoglycemic episode I would not cooperate. So my wife put honey on my lips, which eventually saved me. Each day let's think about helping others.

God's wisdom applies in the following way: to think about what we do. *"The wisdom of the prudent is to give thought to their ways...The prudent see danger and take refuge"* (Proverbs 14:8, 22:3). A great precaution we all can take is to check our blood glucose more often. The other practice is to keep focused on helping others. Not only will they benefit, but we will too!

> **"Two are better than one, because they have a good return for their labor: If either of them falls down, one can help the other up. But pity anyone who falls and has no one to help them up"** —Ecclesiastes 4:9-10.

Remember when you were in school? Were you comfortable sitting with your friends at lunchtime? Or, do you remember lunchtime being a time you dreaded because you sat alone? Sitting by yourself is lonely and uncomfortable, especially when everyone else seems to be laughing and enjoying the company of friends. How many new kids sitting alone may think they are the objects of laughter?

Long ago, I heard a professor share this interesting saying: "It's not what I think that's important; it's not what you think that is important, but it's what I think you think that's important." There are usually no lunchtime welcoming committees for new kids! Most students or teenagers show little concern about new people. *"A person who isn't friendly looks out only for himself"* (Proverbs 18:1). How true that proverb is at lunchtime in many schools.

At Boca High School in Florida, the "We Dine Together" group abruptly halted an ordinary lunchtime. Denis Estimon and three other students began the year determined not to let anyone eat alone unless they wanted to. This started during Denis's senior year, but he remembered being lonely as an immigrant first-grader. Dozens are now members of a high school of 3,400 students. Other schools have initiated "We Dine Together" clubs.[58] Those in their 50s who remember how it was growing up are expressing their comments of appreciation for what they are doing. They told their appreciation with such comments as "lunch periods were achingly uncomfortable" or "I walked instead of ate lunch." One mother discovered her son suffered so much social isolation that he would hide while eating.

What would Jesus do? He taught, *"Do to others as you would have them do to you"* (Luke 6:31). Jesus reached out to socially isolated people—lepers, tax collectors, and the sick. He even ate with tax collectors, who were avoided and ridiculed by others. Jesus knew kindness and attention were greatly appreciated. Paul wrote, *"Always try to be kind to each other and to everyone else...clothe yourselves with compassion, kindness, humility, gentleness and patience...whoever refreshes others will be refreshed... goodwill is found among the upright"* (1 Thessalonians 5:15, Colossians 3:12, Proverbs 11:25, 14:9).

These teenagers are practicing God's wisdom in a wonderfully kind way! "We Dine Together" clubs run in every state and even Canada.

Watch: "So no student eats alone" at https://www.youtube.com/watch?v=IfII5Rw6dBQ and https://www.facebook.com/wedinetogether/

Let's not let others suffer alone. Let's support others because God is helping us with his wisdom. I started a Diabetes Education and Support group in the fall of 1992 and continue to start one wherever I live. God gives us tremendous power through his wisdom to overcome, be resilient, and persevere even with Diabetes and illness! So, let's help others; as we do so, we help ourselves! *"The wise prevail through great power, and those who have knowledge muster their strength...For the LORD gives wisdom; from his mouth come knowledge and understanding. He holds success in store for the upright... Do not let them out of your sight, keep them within your heart; for they are life to those who find them and health to one's whole body"* (Proverbs 24:5, 2:7-8, 4:21-22).

Part 2
Common Sense Guidelines
for Living Well with Diabetes

CHAPTER FOUR

Be Motivated

"I'm discouraged, feel lousy, and just can't seem to do what I need to do." Do you ever experience feelings like that? Yet, motivation is needed to walk more, count carbohydrates, check blood sugar, and avoid foods that drive up blood sugar. What motivates you?

Does avoiding long-term diabetes complications like blindness, amputation, foot pain from peripheral neuropathy, kidney failure, and heart disease motivate you to conquer diabetes? Does that fear motivate you to "go get it done" to control your blood sugars today? Or are you like I thought? Complications are what other people experience, not me. Besides, the possibilities of complications are in the distant future, not today.

When looking at the challenges of controlling diabetes, why not focus on feeling better today? If I feel better today, I can avoid or lower the risk of complications, help others do the same, look and be healthy, continue to enjoy the company of those I love—friends, family, and grandchildren, and do the right things by developing healthy habits!

The following quote is uplifting because it speaks of the expectation of success. *"For the LORD gives wisdom; from his mouth come knowledge and understanding. He holds success (or victory) in store for the upright"* (Proverbs 2:7-8). So, when I do everything needed to outsmart diabetes with this resource, success will be the result. That is motivational; it helps us focus on the goal of victory. And God gives his wisdom for us to succeed, to have victory for health and wellness. God cares about us! *"My son, pay attention to what I say; turn your ear to my words. Do not let them out of your sight, keep them within your heart; for they are life to those who find them and **health to one's whole body"*** (Proverbs 4:20-22).

I included seventeen wise ways to outsmart diabetes from the resource of God's wisdom. They are common-sense approaches for everything needed to manage this disease that is under-rated, insidious, but deadly. The following example shows the importance of motivation after a horrendous accident. It is the kind of motivation we can all practice.

After Tragedy

Facing tragedy is difficult, especially because it could change everything about a person's life. This happened to a Mayo Clinic ER Doctor. As he was biking with a friend and riding over a hill, the next thing he knew, he was looking up at a group of concerned people. He had a strange numb feeling around his waist. When he tried to move his legs, they wouldn't respond. He spent the next four and a half months learning wheelchair basics, like how to get in and out of his wheelchair without falling.

After this disaster, he knew of only two choices about what

he would do with his life. He knew he was going to do something about his paralysis, or he was going to sit and wallow in self-pity. He chose the first and was back at work five months after the accident.

This doctor believes being in a wheelchair has made him a better physician. He would tower over people with his six-foot, five-inch height, but now he is on their level. He thinks his conversations have become much more understanding with patients. For example, he has a typical patient-doctor interaction when he asks questions and orders blood work. Then he pulls back the curtain and reveals that both the patient and doctor are in wheelchairs.

What drives him on? Being a physician is what he's always wanted to be. He smiles and considers it his privilege to practice medicine and to help influence the lives of others. He knows he could have died.[59]

We see in the story of Doctor David Grossman how important having the attitude to overcome obstacles is. God's wisdom states, *"If you are wise, your wisdom will reward you"* (Proverbs 9:12). How was God's wisdom rewarding him? He didn't give up. He had the attitude to overcome. *"The spirit of a man will sustain him in sickness, but who can bear a broken spirit?"* (Proverbs 18:14 NKJV). We also see how valuable compassionately relating to others is. Peter wrote in his first letter, *"Finally, all of you, be like-minded, **be sympathetic**, love one another, be **compassionate and humble**"* (1 Peter 3:8).

As I read this story, I thought about how understanding Jesus, our great physician, is with us. Jesus not only knew about the struggles and hardships people face, but **he experienced**

them himself. The author of Hebrews wrote, *"Although Jesus was the Son [of God], he learned to be obedient **through his sufferings"*** (Hebrews 5:8). The good news is God gives us his wisdom to overcome tragedy and have victory in life (Read Proverbs 2:6-7). Watch "ER Physician Forms Stronger Bond with Patients after Tragedy | NBC Nightly News" at https://www.youtube.com/watch?v=gaV4tsrc_JA

CHAPTER FIVE

Use God's Wisdom
More Valuable than Rubies

A man was stunned and overjoyed when an appraiser valued his blanket at an Antique Roadshow. The blanket is considered one of the Roadshow's "Greatest Finds!" The episode starts with an appraiser, Donald Ellis asking the owner to tell him what he knows about the blanket. He didn't know much except that Kit Carson was supposed to have given it to the foster father of his grandmother. He thought it was a Navajo blanket and had never had it appraised. "Ted, did you notice that when you showed this to me, I stopped breathing a little bit," said the appraiser. "It's a chief's blanket, a Ute First Phase wearing blanket. The Navajo's made it from about 1840 to 1860. They were very valuable at that time. This is Navajo weaving in its purest form." Then he was told its condition was "unbelievable."

He had seen nothing so important on the Roadshow. Ted did not have a clue about its value. He was then asked, "Are you a wealthy man?" No! A shocked, overwhelming reaction followed when he told him its value. "On a really bad day, this blanket would be worth 350,000 dollars and on a good day a half-million dollars." Ted was stunned! If Kit Carson owned it, he said its value would increase by 20%. Ted then became so emotional that he began to gasp for air. He was flabbergasted, knowing his grandparents were just poor farmers. Some of his last words were, "Thank you!" Almost a half-million views have been recorded of this episode on YouTube. Some comments are, "This one really pulls on the heartstrings," or "his reaction is priceless! Congratulations, Sir!"

The blanket was just lying at Ted's home. We have something more valuable than rubies lying at home! What is it? Wisdom, God's word! *"Blessed are those who find wisdom, those who gain understanding.... She is more precious than rubies; nothing you desire can compare with her"* (Proverbs 3:13-15). The good news is we can use it! *"Through wisdom your days will be many, and years will be added to your life. If you are wise, your wisdom will reward you"* (Proverbs 9:11-12). This is a priceless resource that God is providing for our use! *"Trust in the LORD with all your heart and lean not on your own understanding; in all your ways acknowledge him, and he will make your paths straight"* (Proverbs 3:5-6). "Trust" is a concept that includes the idea of safety, confidence, and security. Following God's wisdom creates a sense of security and safety. His wisdom makes life straight, bringing safety, security, confidence, and better health. Learning to acknowledge God and his wisdom in a wide variety of different situations gives us hope. We have something more valuable than rubies or a Navajo Ute chief's blanket!

Watch at: "Top Finds: Mid-19th Century Navajo Ute First Phase Blanket" https://www.youtube.com/watch?v=WJw2qCnhea0

So, to have a great day, use the following specific insights and "Way of Wisdom" principles to outsmart diabetes. Remember these proverbs from God *"are life to those who find them and **health to one's whole body"** (Proverbs 4:22).

"The Road to Good Health Is Always Under Construction. When You Are Through Learning, You Are Through. Keep Learning!"

"Those who cherish understanding will soon prosper" (Proverbs 19:8).

"The heart of the discerning acquires knowledge; the ears of the wise seek it out" (Proverbs 18:15).

"A wise man has great power. A man who has knowledge increases his strength" (Proverbs 24:5 NIrV).

Many things occupy our time. We may be doing those things right, but are they the things that will contribute to our well-being? If you've read this far, you must be among the discerning who will cherish understanding and prosper. The following story will illustrate the importance of the 17 wise ways to outsmart diabetes. They are more important than doing things right; they are doing the right things! Daily doing them brings safety in managing and outsmarting diabetes like this example that illustrates essentials.

Safety

*"The wicked flee though no one pursues, but the righteous are as **bold** as a lion"* (Proverbs 28:1). We see a contrast pictured in

this verse. Some are afraid and fleeing or fearing being caught without any sense of security. The others, who are righteous, are secure, safe, and confident and are described as being as bold as a lion.

A sense of security is essential, as evidenced by what happened to a hang glider. On his first day of vacation in Switzerland, one person wanted to see the picturesque scenery. Hang gliding off a 4,000-foot ledge was his idea for doing so. Since he had never hang-glided, he hired a pilot. Stepping off the ledge, he realized the pilot had made a critical error—double-checking his safety harness to make sure it was attached to the glider. Carpenters have a rule—measure twice, cut once. They didn't do that. We can see the terrifying crisis that followed because a camera was attached to the glider. The passenger desperately tried to stay alive as he quickly grabbed the pilot's side. He hung onto his side, then reached for the gliding bar with his left hand. The pilot maneuvers the glider with one hand as he holds onto his passenger with his left hand. He eventually puts his left hand on his passenger's left hand for more support.

After one hundred thirty-four seconds of frightening terror, he lets go. By then, they were so close to the ground he landed and only broke his wrist. When he first looked down over a hundred seconds before, he knew this was it—he wouldn't survive. He kept his grip with all his might, not realizing how hard he gripped until later discovering he had torn his left bicep.[60]

People want security and safety in life, which builds their confidence. So many people, however, are going through life like the man whose harness was unattached. They experience one crisis after another. Remember where we started with people fleeing and the others being as bold as a lion? The Hebrew word for "Bold" is often translated as trust and means safety, security, and confidence. The word is used ten times in the Proverbs. Another passage tells us how to have this boldness and confidence. This passage teaches how to have a safety harness attached for security in this life. The teaching is to practice wisdom; by doing so, we trust in God. *"Whoever gives heed to instruction prospers, and blessed is the one who **trusts** in the LORD"* Proverbs 16:20.

Let's heed planning and careful consideration of what we do: *"The simple believe anything, but the prudent give thought to their steps...The plans of the diligent lead to profit as surely as haste leads to poverty"* Proverbs 14:15, 21:5. He says he will hang glide again because he "did not get to enjoy my first flight." What do you think will happen with his safety harness?

Watch: "SWISS MISHAP" at https://www.youtube.com/watch?v=dLBJA8SIH2w&t=163s

CHAPTER SIX

Practice the Essentials

A dditional information on #1 Keep learning and #2 Have a health routine—a plan with patience, perseverance.

I've read, "You cannot underestimate the unimportance of practically everything." Or "Things which matter most must never be put at the mercy of things which matter least." So many people's lives are cluttered with trivial things that contribute nothing to health and well-being. The 17 wise ways we just examined are the vital few, the essentials for outsmarting diabetes. My brother, a former mathematics professor, says, "17 as a prime number is one of the basic building blocks of whole numbers in mathematics." So, also, are these 17 guidelines basic building blocks for outsmarting diabetes and living well? Using these 17 wise ways for over thirty years, I've maintained an A1c of 5.9—6.3 with only a few exceptions (like my worst result of 6.9 once). I only mention this to let you know how beneficial and effective these wise "common sense" guidelines are.

What should your blood glucose average be? One hundred forty or less, which is an A1c of 6.5 percent or less, according to the American Association of Clinical Endocrinologists; or 7.0 percent or less is what it should be, according to the American

Diabetes Association, which is 154 average. A normal A1c is considered 5.6 percent or less.

There is also a concept called the 80/20 principle that has validity. It is the idea that about 80 percent of results come from 20 percent of our actions. We had a peach seedling sprout up in the ground. We put it in a pot and nurtured it until it became big enough to plant in the yard. So, we planted this tiny tree in good soil and watered it occasionally. This nurturing continued after each winter for four years until, in the fifth year, we had a peach tree overflowing with branches burdened with lush, delicious peaches. From a tiny tree, only a few actions brought about more peaches than we can eat. This concept of just a few actions resulting in an abundant harvest Proverbs 27:23-27 explains with an agricultural picture for life or a metaphor for wise management. *("For they*—teachings for skillful living—*are life to those who find them and health to one's whole body"* Proverbs 4:22.)

"Be sure you know the condition of your flocks; give careful attention to your herds." When we do this, what benefits do we see? Few of us have flocks or herds, but we all have a body that we need to manage for health with a proper lifestyle. A motivating reason is stated: *"for riches do not endure forever, and a crown is not secure for all generations."* Work is necessary to have the income to live. Stress is elevated by this income, resulting in an unhealthy situation for the mind and body.

Beautiful benefits accrue if knowing and careful attention is given daily to work or our health. *"When the hay is removed, and new growth appears, and the grass from the hills is gathered in, the lambs will provide you with clothing and the goats with the price of a field. You will have plenty of goats' milk to feed your family"* (Proverbs 27:23-27).

The following true stories in the news and from the history of diabetes management will show how effective these wise ways are for success in dealing with diabetes, other chronic diseases, or any challenge you may face in life. These wise "common sense" principles in these uplifting, true stories will reinforce their use in your life. Some of their benefits don't happen overnight. They accumulate with weeks, months, and years of use. That is why I'm giving examples of patience, perseverance, and planning in the following stories.

Great Understanding

An officer couldn't believe the nerve of a pedestrian walking down the highway at a snail's pace at one mile per hour. The pedestrian had no business even being on the highway. He must have been a hundred years old. The officer even talked to him, but the guy just snapped back at him. This officer was not going to leave him alone on the highway. Therefore, he escorted him until he exited the road. Who was this pedestrian? A tortoise![61]

"Annoyingly frustrated" is a good description of people stuck behind a slow highway driver. At such times, everyone needs the great virtue of patience. Paul placed patience as the first virtue he lists as an attribute of love. *"Love is patient; love is kind"* (1 Corinthians 13:4).

Proverbs 14:29 states, *"Whoever is patient has great understanding, but one who is quick-tempered displays folly."* Jumping to conclusions would have been easy to do with the highway walker, but we read to the end of the story with some patience.

Then we don't have to assume; we understand that the walker was a tortoise. If we give ourselves time to be patient, we can have a greater understanding. We begin to see the whole picture.

Have a health routine—a plan.

Patience: Giving your plan time to work

"Whoever is patient has great understanding, but one who is quick-tempered displays folly" (Proverbs 14:29). Anger (or being quick-tempered) excludes different possibilities and positive results. Folly results from having a "short-fuse" with no time allotted for better choices, seeing things differently, and understanding better. *"Blessed are those who find wisdom, those who gain understanding"* (Proverbs 3:13). Solomon described what understanding brings—long life with honor, value, pleasant ways, peace, and happy life. *"With patience you can convince a ruler, and a gentle word can get through to the hard-headed"* (Proverbs 25:15). Through patience, you gain great understanding and persuade people. Patience means not giving up but continuing to try! Patience is so important, for through patience, you can convince people. How much time should you give to a difficult situation? Consider that giving time to concerns like diabetes management brings understanding; as in the following cases, it brings life itself. The following three stories concerning two thirteen-year-old teenagers and one fourteen-year-old demonstrate the importance of patience and not giving up.

I told the story in my book "The Way of Wisdom for Diabetes" about the first American who received insulin after Frederick

Banting and Charles Best discovered insulin in 1921. His name was James Havens.

The Story of James Havens: The First American to Receive Insulin

It was about Thanksgiving, 1914 when James Havens was diagnosed with what we today call Type 1 diabetes. He was almost fifteen years old. From that day on, the wisdom principle of planning ahead was intensely used for him. During the next seven-and-a-half years planning was necessary to just keep him alive. He continued to plan the next thirty-eight years until he died, not of diabetes, but colon cancer! The idea of planning, of deciding ahead of time what to do, was followed by his mother, for she meticulously planned his meals, weighing every morsel of food he ate.

He was a very fortunate person, as he became the first American to receive insulin. Before insulin, the only therapy was Dr. Frederick Allen's "under-nutrition therapy." Dr. Allen advocated serious dieting to patients, whose complaints were their extreme hunger and rapid weight loss. The doctor seemed to be telling them that they needed to be hungry more often to keep blood sugar levels from skyrocketing higher, eventually leading to coma. Jim endured this for almost eight years until he received insulin. Insulin was discovered in the summer of 1921.

When Jim was diagnosed, he was almost fifteen years old and weighed ninety-seven pounds. From Thanksgiving, 1914, to May 21, 1922, he went from ninety-seven pounds to less than seventy-four pounds. During that time, he endured a meal plan of about 820 calories per day, with painstaking efforts to eliminate most carbohydrates from his meal plan.[62] Deciding ahead of time was required. By doing this, he lived longer than anyone else on this "under-nutrition therapy."

His dad looked and inquired about any new treatments; treatments that would keep his son alive. He was the head of the legal department at the Eastman Kodak Company in Rochester, New York. He searched the United States for eight years, looking for a promising treatment, but none was found. In fact, in March of 1921, his father wrote, "His condition is not such as to hold out any hope."[63]

One day George Snowball, a manager of the Kodak store in Toronto, Canada, came into his office. Mr. Havens asked if he knew anyone in Canada who was working on a cure for diabetes. He didn't, but he would inquire when he got back home. This man began to ask and ask and eventually discovered that Dr. Banting and his assistant, Charles Best, had made an important discovery at the University of Toronto. Of course, it was *insulin*. When Jim's dad received this exciting news, he persuaded his son's doctor, John Williams, to go to Toronto. While there, Williams was able to get some insulin from Dr. Banting.

By May 1922, the only thing Jim could do was moan with excruciating pain. He was barely able to lift his head from his pillow. He was ready for his life to end. In fact, on his hospital chart, it was recorded that he was "anxious to die and end his misery."[64] He could bear it no longer. Over the next few days, his whole outlook was in for a dramatic change. Dr. Williams was able to bring to Rochester a small amount of unrefined insulin. On the evening of May 21, injections of insulin were started, but they seemed to have no affect.

The next week, George Snowball stopped in to see Jim's dad at Eastman Kodak. When he asked about how Jim was doing, he was surprised to hear his dad say, "I guess we're through." "But those fellows have saved lives," Snowball said.[65] Suddenly Mr. Havens shot up out of his seat and said, "George, get one of those young men over here." Mr. Snowball went to Dr. Banting and pleaded with him to go to New York, but he refused. He refused until Snowball said, "The Havens' physician tried your preparation, and it didn't work. They think it's just another failure."

Dr. Banting went to Rochester, and this time Jim received larger doses of insulin. They gave them in two-hour intervals, checking the urine for sugar at each interval. Eventually, after several doses, they all had a euphoric reaction—no sugar was in the urine. The insulin was working! James wrote to Dr. Banting, the discoverer of insulin: "A week ago last Thursday....Marked an historical event as I then tasted my first egg and toast. Egg on toast is my idea of the only food necessary in heaven."

"A cheerful look brings joy to your heart. And good news gives health to your body" (Proverbs 15:30 NIrV). We can be thankful today that we don't have to endure what James Havens had to face. His comment after receiving insulin was a comment of gratitude! When I realize we have so many new resources available today like glucose meters, new types of insulin, insulin pumps and pens, and an assortment of medications, and other ways to prevent or cope with complications that weren't available more than fifty years ago, I am overwhelmed with gratitude! I believe this gratitude perspective can help anyone face the challenge to outsmart diabetes when used daily.

For more than seven years, James Havens persevered with

the support of his parents. With patience and perseverance, his life was saved. He continued to plan his meals and take daily injections of insulin for the rest of his life. If he hadn't been one of the fortunate ones at that time his life would have been over. Instead, he lived another thirty-eight years. We never know what wonderful results will appear when we persevere with patience and planning. We too have access to these powerful principles of planning, perseverance, and patience. *"Do not those who plot evil go astray? But those who plan what is good find love and faithfulness...Sluggards do not plow in season; so at harvest time they look but find nothing...The plans of the diligent lead to profit as surely as haste leads to poverty"* (Proverbs 14:22, 20:4, 21:5). As a result, we'll be rewarded for using them, which will then reinforce their repeated use in our lives.

A Freak Accident

Thirteen-year-old Trenton was in a freak accident. His friend was driving a utility vehicle and pulling him in an attached wagon. He came around a corner too fast and flipped the wagon. Trenton's head hit the ground, and the wagon landed on his head, causing seven skull fractures. After being rushed to the hospital, a doctor admitted he had "no brain waves, a damaged brain stem, and his heart only beat because of adrenaline." He was in a coma and on life support in the hospital. If he were to regain consciousness, he would be like a vegetable.

His future looked bleak. After weeks in this condition, his parents signed papers to donate Trenton's organs to five children. The day before his doctors scheduled his life support to end, he moved his fingers and then a foot and regained consciousness.

Soon Trenton was shooting baskets from his wheelchair in the hospital gym. His mom said he is healing daily; she praises the Lord for his recovery. He has his full memory. He talks about his school friends. His healing continues now at home.[66]

Have you ever heard anyone answer "how are you" with "hanging in there?" I usually say, "don't let go." God's wisdom says, *"Whoever is patient has great understanding"* (Proverbs 14:29). Keep hanging on with patience because patience gives an understanding that healing takes time. Have you ever done physical therapy for weeks with no results, and then suddenly, the treatment begins to work? If you ever need patience under challenging circumstances, remember Proverbs 14:29! Just quote it. You will be surprised at how helpful the repeating of God's wisdom is.

Watch: Miracle Boy' Trenton McKinley Wakes From Coma Just Before Organ Harvesting | TODAY at **https://www.youtube.com/watch?v=Krpdx6YyCTA**

"Love is patient. Love is kind" 1 Corinthians 13:4.

Here is another example of patience and an optimistic attitude.

783 Days

A recent human-interest story concerned a thirteen-year-old girl who needed a heart transplant. After being on the transplant list for 783 days, she was scheduled to get a pacemaker, not a heart. They had not found an available heart, and her health had worsened so that she couldn't wait any longer. Anna's zest for life, her desire, and her optimism were never a concern; instead, it was the problem with her heart.

The transplant team had scheduled her to be at Texas Children's Hospital at six in the morning, and her mother said, "They were short on beds." She was beginning to wonder if it was even going to happen. Four hours later, nurses were finally prepping Anna for her surgery. Anna even got the IV. But then there was more waiting. The family wondered if they had gone to lunch and forgotten about Anna. They sat for another hour and a half. Finally, Anna's transplant coordinator entered the room with several other people. They said, "Anna, are you excited about getting your ICD (implantable cardioverter-defibrillator) today?" She said, "I guess so," and the coordinator said, "How would you like a new heart instead?"

One week after receiving a new heart, she became stronger daily, walking, talking, and smiling. The family concluded that if the initially scheduled surgery had happened on time, the donor heart for which they had waited 783 days would have gone to someone else. The delay saved her that day![67]

God's wisdom is aptly seen in this beautiful story too. How? We see the value of patience, an optimistic attitude, and perseverance all on display! It's evident from this story that patience does carry a lot of wait. Too many people are not willing to wait. She wouldn't have experienced a new heart if she had given up. We can grasp the full meaning of the proverb that *"Those who are patient have great understanding"* (Proverbs 14:29). She could understand the value in staying optimistic, not giving up and waiting day in and day out for 783 days because they are what brought her to the point of receiving a new heart! Her optimistic attitude sustained her through this sickness. *"The will to live can get you through sickness, but no one can live with a broken spirit"* (Proverbs 18:14 NCV). The temptation is to expect quick results, but the wise thing to do is stay patient and optimistic and trust God and his wisdom. *"Eat honey, my son, for it is good; honey from the comb is sweet to your taste. Know also that wisdom is sweet to your soul; if you find it, there is a future hope for you, and your hope will not be cut off"* (Proverbs 24:13-14).

How to Live with Diabetes When Doctors Diagnosed Me as a Seven-Year-Old in 1960

With all the resources available today, you are now living in the best of times to outsmart diabetes. Add to the resources the principles of God's wisdom, like gratitude, patience, perseverance, and discernment, and you can succeed! When I was diagnosed with diabetes in December of 1960, the book "How to Live with Diabetes" by Henry Dolger, M.D. was given to me (Dr. Dolger was the Distinguished Chief of The Medical Staff of the Mount Sinai Diabetes Clinic, New York City). Very little was known about diabetes then compared to what is known today.

There was only one oral medication when this book was written. The medication was called Orinase. Dr. Dolger wrote, "Where the patients were between 20 and 40, Orinase was effective in four out of five cases. In juvenile diabetes and where the patients were under 20, Orinase was rarely effective. Also, he writes, "There is no relation to the length of time a person has had diabetes and his response to Orinase. Long-standing cases showed good response, as did new cases. Nor was the body type of the patient a factor in response to Orinase." He continued,

"Clearly, for a large number of diabetics, Orinase presaged a revolution in treatment virtually as great as that brought about by the discovery of insulin."[68] There were several theories given as to why it worked, but the right one was the stimulation of the pancreas to secrete insulin.

Now medications are available that use incretin hormones like Ozempic and Mounjaro, DPP4 enzyme inhibitors, slow down the digestive system, prevent the release of stored glucose or glycogen in the liver and others that help with blood glucose control in the kidneys independent of insulin. There are injectable combinations of these medications that are injected daily or just once a week.

When I was first diagnosed about sixty years ago, only thick hypodermic needles were used. Dr. Dolger wrote, "It should be 25 to 26 gauge. A reserve supply of needles should always be kept on hand because needles may bend or break and, in any case, usually become dull after about two weeks' use."[69] I remember those needles becoming dull and very uncomfortable with each painful injection. Today we use insulin pens or syringes with ultra-thin needles with gauges of 31 or 32. Yes, we've come to a much better day for living well. So, keep working on control with patience, perseverance, and knowledgeable judgment of what to do each day, and you, too, will succeed.

CHAPTER SEVEN

Stay Positive with Gratitude for Living Well

(Additional information on #6—Focus on staying positive every day with gratitude.)

S cientific research on gratitude has demonstrated many incredible benefits. Benefits include being more optimistic, connected with others, sleeping better, being more compliant in following a meal and exercise plan, and taking medicine. These benefits also reduce stress, decreasing levels of counterregulatory hormones like epinephrine (adrenaline) and cortisol that cause insulin resistance and elevated blood glucose. Here are stories that illustrate and reinforce the practice of gratitude.

Positive Focus

"A cheerful heart is good medicine, but a crushed spirit dries up the bones" (Proverbs 17:22). A cheerful heart is good medicine. Laughter, smiles, and even tears came to a family when their baby daughter heard her older sister for the first time after she received hearing aids. The older sister kept saying, "Baby sister, baby sister," and then the baby sister began to giggle and laugh.

Laughing and laughing, she started jumping up and down on her mother's knee as her older sister continued to talk to her. Gasping with joy, the mother covered her mouth. She could not contain her tears of joy. Smiling and looking up at her mom, she pauses and then breaks out with laughter again as she looks at her sister. The whole scene displayed the truth of the proverb that a cheerful heart is good medicine! Why do scenes like that bring joy to all of us? The reason is we like good news. This was certainly good news for the baby and her family! *"A cheerful look brings joy to your heart. And good news gives health to your body"* (Proverbs 15:30). When people are diagnosed with diabetes, lifestyle changes need to happen. So, we shouldn't fear change because, as this story illustrates, good news in one's life and well-being can result!

> **Watch:** "Adorable: Baby's Reaction Hearing New Sounds with Help of Hearing Aid" at **https://www.youtube.com/ watch?v=hgjC68KOjSQ**

Here is another beautiful good news story. Standing in a grocery checkout line is often frustrating, especially if yours is just slowly moving. What if you were waiting and then realizing you forgot your billfold? This happened to an older man one day. His frustration and alarm turned into good news, as the person ahead of him was an observant young woman who offered to pay for his groceries. He was very appreciative, wanted to pay her back, and asked for her mailing address. Sure enough, a few days later, she received a fifteen-dollar check with this note. "You saved me a lot of trouble. My wife is ill, and I wanted to get back to her. I'm not very young anymore—84 years old. It's not a surprise I left my wallet at home. I shall always remember your kindness." This was good news for the man and the young woman. She doesn't plan to cash the check. She says, "I have something that I look at every morning when I leave my room. It says 'be the reason that someone smiles today' so I see that when I leave my house. That was what I could do to make him smile that day."[70]

Stories like these build goodwill and gratitude in life. I'm thankful I saw the video and could read the notes from the incident at the grocery store. Positive stories like these are where God's wisdom directs us. *"He who seeks good finds goodwill, but evil comes to him who searches for it"* (Proverbs 11:27).

"If You're Happy and You Know It . . ."

"A happy heart makes the face cheerful, but heartache crushes the spirit...All the days of the oppressed are wretched, but the cheerful heart has a continual feast" (Proverbs 15:13, 15). What contributes to a continuous cheerful feast? We must keep pumping in the air to keep a leaky tire from going flat. To keep a cheerful heart from falling into the gloomy depths of dreariness, we must keep pumping the heart with thoughts from the brighter side of life! Some of these ideas are not only good but can be humorous as well.

For example, let Phoebe, who is a Cockatiel, cheer us. I heard Phoebe chirping the opening tune of "If You're Happy and You Know It." The next phrase is "Clap your hands." Since she has no hands, she uses her beak to tap on a banana or the table to "clap your hands." She enthusiastically continues to do this for over a minute, building up to a final crescendo. When you click on this link, "Bird Sings If You're Happy and You Know It ‖ ViralHog" at https://www.youtube.com/watch?v=zFxwNlccSt4, you, too, will be clapping your hands!

Stay Fresh and Green

Another encouraging story is the story of Dr. Robert Moore. This San Jose man's 100th birthday celebration went to the dogs last Saturday. Literally! The family decided to honor their father, who loves dogs and is known as a dog whisperer, by having a parade of dogs in front of his house so he could pet them. Those who wanted to wish him happy birthday were to come with their dogs dressed in cowboy hats, or tuxedos, and so on. They put the notice on the Nextdoor app expecting maybe twenty to thirty dogs. To their surprise, more than two hundred dogs came! The line extended around the block and down the street, for there were so many. There were pups with disabilities, dogs pulling carts, and even canines in classic cars. Dr. Robert Moore, former dean at San Jose State University, with his avid love of dogs, demonstrated it that day by petting each one who came and thanking the owners of each dog!

The Moore family was heartened by how the community came with their dogs and brought him flowers, cupcakes, drawings, and posters. His daughter said, "My father, he was so touched. He pet every single dog that came through. Every person brought the dog up to him. It was so lovely." Yes, even at 100, I see his fresh and green attitude, as the psalmist expressed. *"The righteous will flourish like a palm tree, they will grow like a cedar of Lebanon; planted in the house of the LORD, they will flourish in the courts of our God. They will still bear fruit in old age, they will stay fresh and green, proclaiming, 'The LORD is upright; he is my Rock, and there is no wickedness in him'"* Psalm 92:12-15. Let's all strive to have that attitude each day!

Focusing on stories like this is the practice of **God's wisdom.** *"He who seeks good finds goodwill, but evil comes to him who searches for it"* (Proverbs 11:27). It is meaningful that Proverbs 17:22 states, *"a cheerful heart is good medicine."* By reading these stories and watching Phoebe, the Cockatiel, we will experience the good medicine that brings a cheerful heart. *"A cheerful look brings joy to your heart. And good news gives health to your body"* (Proverbs 15:30).

"How good is a timely word" (Proverbs 15:23).

"A word fitly spoken is like apples of gold in a setting of silver" (Proverbs 25:11). One word can make a difference in a person's life. One word made the difference for a soldier in the Vietnam War almost fifty years ago. What was that word? Was it love, compassion, kindness, or gentleness? No, although it expressed those ideas, "thanks" was the word.

A sixth-grade girl completed her homework assignment with "thanks." She sent a letter of encouragement to a soldier—a soldier she did not even know! John has kept this note ever since he received it for Christmas 1970. Following is the message sent to him: "Dear Serviceman, I want to give my sincere thanks for going over to war to fight for us. The class hopes you will be able to come home."

"Thanks" is a powerful word of appreciation that is sparingly used. Remember when Jesus healed the ten lepers how many came back to him and said thanks? Yes, only one came back and used that word to thank him.

Any soldier could have received the girl's note, but John appreciated it. His job was dangerous on a helicopter each day. He said, "When you got up in the morning, you always wondered whether you would see the sun go down at night." He still has the note hidden behind a picture in his living room.

John's family found DonnaCaye, the sixth-grade girl who wrote the thankful message. They even arranged a surprise meeting. When he saw her, he exclaimed, "You're real." "I'm real," DonnaCaye said, and "I remember writing the letter. I was amazed that I could have the opportunity to write to a serviceman and maybe make his life a little simpler for a couple of minutes." Her word of "thanks" has continued to help past those first minutes. The words have continued to encourage him for almost fifty years. "Fact is, I think it means more today than it did when I got it," John admitted. He received thanks; he still treasures it![71]

Words have power as the proverb says. *"What you say can mean life or death. Those who speak with care will be rewarded"* (Proverbs 18:21 NCV). We see from this note that both were rewarded! The apostle Paul writes, *"and be thankful...give thanks in all circumstances for this is God's will for you in Christ Jesus"* (Colossians 3:15, 1 Thessalonians 5:18).

Positive Notes

An artist leaves positive notes to strangers. His purpose is to brighten up their day. He does this in South London. He's been doing this for three years. He relates he used to work in advertising, but he became sick and discouraged. He was off work for a month. When he returned he had a long commute to work. So, he decided to hopefully make a difference to at least one person a day by posting positive notes. Any feedback could be sent to Instagram Notes to Strangers. Strangers began writing back in appreciation for his messages. He was making a difference! After posting these positive notes for nine months it became his full-time job. It's from a variety of places that he gets his sayings like "You can always start again" or "Your best friend was once a stranger" or "Kindness spreads." His notes are popping up in The Alps, Amsterdam, Paris, Florida, and California.

Some people are looking at the sayings he's posting and are being influenced in a positive way. *"Pleasant words are like honey. They are sweet to the spirit and bring healing to the body"* (Proverbs 16:24). It has been said, "Sow a thought, reap an action. Sow an action, reap a habit. Sow a habit, reap a character. Sow a character, reap a destiny." This makes our thinking so important. Proverbs 4:23 says, *"Be careful what you think, because your thoughts run your life"* (NIrV).

Would you like to read words that build your confidence, words that are positive and uplifting, words that are motivational, words that give you a greater sense of hope and well-being? I believe we would all like to read words like that. Consider this--*"Wisdom is sweet to your soul; if you find it, there is a future hope for you, and your hope will not be cut off"* (Proverbs 24:13).

Since God's Wisdom gives us hope; why not use the following words for a prayer. They are the words of Paul's prayer for the church at Colossae. *"May you be made strong with all the strength that comes from his glorious power, and may you be prepared to endure everything with patience, while joyfully giving thanks to the Father"* (Colossians 1:11-12 NRSV). Those words are surely encouraging! When we pray that prayer, God will build our attitudes with confidence. He will give hope in facing difficult challenges as well as endurance with gratitude—*"endure everything... while joyfully giving thanks."* These are pleasant words that bring healing. Let's not only pray such words, but let's use positive words with ourselves and others!

> **"An anxious heart weighs a man down, but a kind word cheers him up" (Proverbs 12:25).**

Watch: "Artist Places Encouraging Post-It Notes Around London | NBC Nightly News" at **https://www.youtube.com/watch?v=RcN11zHhbtI**

New Life

A child's first birthday is a very special occasion! Happiness characterizes these celebrations. The first birthday only happens once in a person's life, but not for Ed. He is different because he has two first birthdays. He could celebrate twice because he was given a second chance for life at the age of sixty-four.

When attending a party to celebrate his oldest son's birthday on September 22, 2013, he became very ill and had to leave. When he got home, he felt worse and was rushed to the hospital. He had lost a great deal of blood. His liver was starting to shut down and his liver problem was compounded with kidney damage as well.

April 3, 2017, was his worst day. He was in the hospital and on kidney dialysis, plus his name was on a transplant list. He remembered telling his wife, "I was giving up, I was done, I was on dialysis, and I was in so much pain." Less than two hours later he got the news that would change his life—surgery tomorrow. On April 4th he received his new organs! "It's fun to be able to take care of these patients in the most exciting time of their life, at the time of transplant and to continue to help them through their recovery," nurse Shelby remarked.[72]

Ed says, "Every day is a great day when I wake up." He expresses how he is constantly thankful. He has a newfound appreciation for birthday celebrations, family get-togethers and holidays. His first birthday was not only a personal celebration but also a fundraiser for the Gift of Life Transplant House near the Mayo Clinic. The house provides a place to stay for both caregivers and those recovering from their transplants. *"A generous person will prosper; whoever refreshes others will be refreshed"* Proverbs 11:25). *"This is the day the Lord has made; We will rejoice and be glad in it"* (Psalm 118:24 NKJV).

A Bag of Money

Making the right decisions about what to do can affect not only the person but also many others. Consider the following proverbs, which show a mixture of good and bad results. The importance of choices like working at the right time, being honest, and showing generosity determine results.

> *"Sluggards do not plow in season; so at harvest time they look but find nothing"* (Proverbs 20:4).

> *"The LORD detests lying lips, but he delights in people who are trustworthy"* (Proverbs 12:22).

> *"The generous will themselves be blessed, for they share their food with the poor"* (Proverbs 22:9).

A community food bank shares food, helping about a thousand people per month. They also take backpacks full of food to school-aged children each Friday, assisting five hundred children so they have food for the weekend. A box outside the food bank entrance is filled with bread three times a day. One morning, twenty minutes before opening, a homeless man looked inside the box and saw a heavy bag sitting there. He opened it and pulled out a twenty-dollar bill. He then looked inside and saw that the bag was full of twenty and hundred-dollar bills— $17,000 in total!

It was decision time. What was he to do? Remember, he is homeless. His decision would determine whether there would be a harvest of help for many or just for him. Would he be honest and kind? Would he turn the bag of money over to the food bank?

Here is what Kevin said. "That was a really big decision for me, but if it's not yours, you shouldn't be taking it. There are a lot of people who would have taken it. I'm just not that person." He waited twenty minutes and turned the bag over to the food bank as it opened that morning. They then turned it over to the police, who did an investigation to try to find the owner of the money. No one claimed it and after ninety days, the money belonged to the food bank. Officers had a ceremony for the food bank, returning the money to it and honoring Kevin for his honesty. "Not every citizen would be as honest as you in this situation," said the officer. In appreciation, the food bank plans periodically to give Kevin gift cards to his favorite store.[73]

Not only was Kevin honest but he was kind. He knew that by turning the money over to the food bank, more people would be helped. The news media focuses on unkindness, dishonesty, and mistreatment of others. Kindness is an important trait that is so often underestimated. How many times do we hear about the kindness of people? Let's make decisions that will result in kind benefits to others.

"What is desirable in a man is his kindness"
Proverbs 19:22 (NASB)

Watch: "Homeless man turns in $17,000 he found outside food bank" at https://www.youtube.com/watch?v=8_tT7WikOZE

CHAPTER EIGHT

Get Up and Move for Living Well

Additional information on #7—Move often throughout Every Day.

I f you were told about a once-a-day pill that could help you sleep better, restore your energy, improve your mood, reduce your risk of heart disease, help you to lose weight, and improve your blood sugar control, you would probably take it in an instant! And movement does all of that! It doesn't even stop there, because it can also increase your good cholesterol (HDL), lower your bad cholesterol (LDL), and improve blood pressure. If you have a gloomy mood, then move more. Movement can stimulate the brain to release endorphins, which are positive mood changers, and also release serotonin, which can stave off depression.[74]

Hard Work

What does God's wisdom say about work? *"Those who work their land will have abundant food, but those who chase fantasies have no sense...From the fruit of their lips people are filled with good things, and the work of their hands brings them reward...All hard work brings a profit, but mere talk leads only to poverty"* (Proverbs

12:11,14, 14:23). Work brings monetary and material rewards, but the common work in 1000 BC, the time these proverbs were written, brought another type of reward. Here is an example of that type of work. *"Let me go to the fields and pick up the leftover grain behind anyone in whose eyes I find favor." Naomi said to her, "Go ahead, my daughter." So she went out, entered a field and began to glean behind the harvesters. As it turned out, she was working in a field belonging to Boaz* (Ruth 2:2-3). This type of work would bring monetary rewards, but this type of work would also bring another type of reward—physical health. Moving, lifting, turning, guiding a plow with an ox, and harvesting a crop by hand would all be common activities then. Images like that would come to people's minds as they thought of these proverbs. Sitting in front of a desk would not enter the mind of the wise, but rather standing and moving jobs would—manual labor!

When thinking about the benefits of work, the following news headline grabbed my attention: "A father and his sons cut wood to fill 80 trucks. Then they brought it to homes that needed heat."[75] That headline was meaningful because these men were not doing this to benefit themselves but rather to help the needy.

At first, this forty-seven-year-old father and his twenty-one-year-old twin sons were chopping together as a family activity. They like to chop wood; it is a family tradition. The father did it with his father and he has passed the tradition on to his sons. Last summer they started chopping and the wood kept accumulating until it reached a value of over 15,000 dollars. In Washington State where they live, 20-degree temperatures were coming in early November. They could easily start selling wood, but instead, they decided to post it as "free" on Facebook and see what would happen. They got request after request from people in real need. They not only gave it away but also during the evenings they would even deliver the wood.

They began bringing wood to hundreds of needy people who do not have money to buy it. They began helping some of the neediest people in their area, who only use wood to heat their homes. One single mom, living in a mobile home with only a wood-burning stove for heat, was overwhelmed with the generosity. She said, "To get that much wood and the chimney sweep brought me to tears. So much stress and anxiety for my daughter is off my shoulders. I couldn't be more thankful."

These three men are often met with tears and hugs of heartfelt gratitude as they make deliveries. The father, Shane McDaniel, said something very insightful, "It has nothing to do with how well it's received, but it's about how much it's needed."

This is an impressive story of hard work and generosity. It reminds me of what Luke wrote about Paul. *"In everything I did, I showed you that by this kind of hard work we must help the weak, remembering the words the Lord Jesus himself said: 'It is more blessed to give than to receive' "* (Acts 20:35).

It is a sin to despise one's neighbor, but blessed is the one who is kind to the needy (Proverbs 14:21).

107 Years and Working Hard

One person allows only one barber to cut his hair because of his experience. He says, "This guy's been cutting hair for a century." That was an exaggeration because he's only been cutting hair for ninety-six years. Mr. Mancinelli started in 1921 when

Warren G. Harding was president. He has cut hair for generations—fathers, grandfathers, great-grandfathers. Some customers have been coming to him for more than fifty years, getting
hundreds of haircuts from just him.[76]

Yes, he has experience starting in 1921 as a boy of about
11 and continuing to this day at 107 years old. Longevity is
what usually happens when people use a wise "common sense"
approach to life. *"Blessed are those who find wisdom... Long life is
in her right hand"* (Proverbs 3:13, 16).

His very example is an inspiration to some of his older
customers. His son relates his favorite phrase for eighty-year-
old customers is "Listen, when you get to be my age..." That's
encouragement, and "they love hearing it." *"Worry weighs a person down; an encouraging word cheers a person up... A cheerful
heart is good medicine, but a crushed spirit dries up the bones"*
(Proverbs 12:25, 17:22).

He works hard, never calls in sick and even sweeps up the
hair clippings himself. He continues to work and keeps busy five
days a week from noon until 8 p.m. He works Saturdays when it
is most busy. A young fellow worker said she gets tired being on
her feet all day "but he just keeps going." *"All hard work brings a
profit, but mere talk leads only to poverty"* (Proverbs 14:23).

To stay busy and work full-time helps him to stay upbeat
after the loss of his wife fourteen years ago. He misses her and
goes to her grave every day before going to work. Loyal is what
he is to his work and as well as to his wife of sixty-nine years.
*"Many claim to have unfailing love, but a faithful person who can
find?"* (Proverbs 20:6).

Many people ask about his secret to longevity and his simple answer is to just put in a satisfying day of work. He also uses a wise "common sense" approach to what he eats, avoiding harmful drinks and foods. He claims he stays thin by eating thin spaghetti. From the way of wisdom, the "common sense" approach to life includes the following: *"From the fruit of their lips people are filled with good things, and the work of their hands brings them reward... Lazy people want much but get little, but those who work hard will prosper... The wisdom of the prudent is to give thought to their ways"* (Proverbs 12:14, 13:4, 14:8). Sounds like a good approach for wise living! Patient, too, with the variety of clients he's had in almost a century. He died on Sept 19, 2019, at his home in New Windsor, N.Y., a Hudson River town about an hour's drive north of New York City. He was 108. His son, Bob, 82, said the cause was jaw cancer. His father had retired, reluctantly, only weeks before. "He didn't know the meaning of the word retired," Bob Mancinelli said. That is being on his feet and being very patient in his work.

Watch: "This 107-Year-Old Is the World's Oldest Barber" at https://www.youtube.com/watch?v=B9jH-3yITAk

Movement Motivation: A Walk to the Hospital

Some people can do amazing things. Walking six miles round trip from home to the hospital would not be surprising for a man in his twenties. To be ninety-nine and walk that distance each day is quite remarkable.

Most people would accept a ride if offered or take the bus. Luther does neither. He's done a lot of walking in his life since his work involved manual labor. He also says the walk clears his mind. Those are not the real motivating factors for his determination to walk to the hospital each day. What motivates him is his love for his wife. They've been married for fifty-five years now, and he doesn't want her to be there by herself. His wife was diagnosed with a brain tumor in 2009. She has been in and out of the hospital; her most current stay has been for three months. Her bedside is where he belongs, and so he walks. On one occasion, a reporter walked with him. As he got closer to the hospital, he even picked up his pace and began to run.[77]

The love for his wife gives him the willpower to walk no matter the weather. His walking is not just because he loves her but also because she loves him. He says, "She's my wife; she's my best friend." When he says walking clears his mind, what remains in his mind is his wife's love for him. Their daughter says, "He's always cared about her the way he does [now]. He loves my mom. He'll do anything for her." This story is not about walking for exercise, although walking is important for health. Luther says he doesn't smoke, doesn't drink. He attributes that to his health also. The love he and his wife have for each other is what makes the difference.

Love is a great motivator. With love, amazing things can happen. The apostle John referred to himself as *"the disciple whom Jesus loved"* (John 21:20). He writes in his first letter *"Dear friends, let us love one another, for love comes from God... Whoever does not love does not know God, because God is love... This is love: not that we loved God, but that he loved us and sent his Son as an atoning sacrifice for our sins. Dear friends, since God so loved us, we also ought to love one another"* (1 John 4:7-8, 10-11). And Solomon writes, *"My son, do not forget my teaching, but keep my commands in your heart, for they will prolong your life many years and bring you peace and prosperity. Let love and faithfulness never leave you; bind them around your neck, write them on the tablet of your heart. Then you will win favor and a good name in the sight of God and man"* (Proverbs 3:1-4).

Watch: 99-Year-Old Walks 6 Miles a Day to Visit His Wife in the Hospital https://www.youtube.com/watch?v=Tb_-PHZO4rE

CHAPTER NINE

Encourage Others for Living Well

*Additional Information on #17—Take advantage
of opportunities to help others.*

To Be Encouraged, Encourage

*"A good person gives life to others; the wise person
teaches others how to live"* (Proverbs 11:30 NCV).

When I was recovering from back surgery, a laminectomy
in 1988, I was kept in a wing of a large hospital just for
patients with diabetes. I was thirty-five. During my stay of ten
days, I discovered five people who were already blind from the
complication of retinopathy; four were younger than me and one
about five years older. It took me almost thirty years to realize
how serious this disease is. I saw it. Two years before this I had a
massive hemorrhage in my right eye. So, I resolved to help people, to help them feel better every day, to support them so that
they wouldn't have to face such devastating complications. That
decision helped me get better control of my diabetes as well.

In the fall of 1992, I started a diabetes support group at the
Good Samaritan Hospital in Kearney, Nebraska. For the first

meeting, thirty-five attended. I introduced myself, and for the next several years, I gave encouraging support to those who attended, helping hundreds of people. For the last twenty-five years, I've continued to facilitate either hospital or community diabetes support groups where ever I've lived.

Many people will not admit they have diabetes or any chronic disease. Their disease is private, their secret. What is missed with that attitude? What is missed is their opportunity to not only help others but to help themselves as well. Eventually the hospital in Kearney, Nebraska hired a Certified Diabetes Educator. One day, I received a call from her, telling me there was a noncompliant patient with Type 1 diabetes in the hospital. Would I visit him? I agreed. He would not cooperate, even putting the sheets over his head when they entered his room. When I asked to enter his room, identifying myself as a fellow Type 1, he invited me in and opened up to me.

We talked about the challenges we were both facing. He was finding great difficulty in keeping his blood sugar under control. He had never had any support or encouragement. His mom was not helpful. Friends of hers had even influenced him to drink. So, after he was released from the hospital, he attended the support group meetings. We also met weekly. I shared portions from a book called "Diabetes: A Guide to Living Well" by Dr. Gary Arsham. Dr. Arsham was diagnosed with Type 1 diabetes when he was ten. Unlike today, there were few books available for people with diabetes in 1994. So, in a sense, he became part of our weekly meetings. People need encouragement. Randy started doing better with his blood sugar levels, but he already had kidney failure. He started on Peritoneal Dialysis.

Not only did we use the diabetes guide book, but we looked at encouraging Proverbs like *"The fear of the LORD is the beginning of wisdom, and knowledge of the Holy One is understanding. For through wisdom your days will be many, and years will be added to your life. If you are wise, your wisdom will reward you"* (Proverbs 9:10-12). He started coming to Bible class. When he started his mom wanted to know why in the world he was doing that. He said because he had never tried it before. He was trying a lot of new things like routinely checking his blood sugar. He wanted to see if attending Bible class would make a difference. And it did!

One day after eating lunch together, as we traveled toward my office, we saw a lawn that really needed mowing. The person who lived there was a widow, a recluse whose husband had died in World War 2. I casually said we should just go mow her lawn. After saying that, I went on a trip out of state. When I got back, I discovered Randy had taken his mower in the trunk of his car and mowed the whole lawn, taking the cuttings to the dump yard. I asked if she ever said anything to him. She only said, "What are you doing?" No, thanks, no gratitude! Randy was practicing God's wisdom. *"Blessed is the one who is kind to the needy"* (Proverbs 14:21). That is the kind of behavior a Christian should have. So, a few days later he became a Christian, being baptized into Christ (read Acts 22:16, Galatians 3:27, Romans 6:3-4).

Randy was on a kidney transplant list, and not long after, this wonderful news arrived—a kidney and pancreas. When he received that pancreas, he was no longer in the community of diabetics. This good news was countered with bad news because within a few weeks, he was in a car/train wreck. The train won.

He was flown to Omaha with a broken femur, ribs, and arm and severe trauma to his head. He was in rehab for months. How did he stay encouraged during those weeks of therapy? He focused on good things. He said just as Paul walked on water, as long as he kept his eyes on Jesus (it was actually Peter), he was encouraged and strengthened. Here is a question he asked me. What is the most rewarding thing about your job? "What is most rewarding," I said, "is when I see people encouraged and helped!"

Look for people you can encourage. For example, start a walking club! One woman at our diabetes support group knew she needed to start walking. She needed motivation! She asked at a support group meeting if anyone would meet her at the park to help her get started. Three people volunteered. But instead of just three showing up, twelve did! Can you imagine how it would be to show up to walk and have about a dozen others there to help you get started? It would be encouraging and motivating! I've discovered that when I look for people I can encourage and support, they've helped me, too! Those who showed up to help her get started walking walked, too. So, in a sense, she was helping them, also. When we look for others to support, we, too, will be encouraged! Being blessed and refreshed will result just as Jesus and Solomon said: *"It is more blessed to give than to receive...A generous person will prosper; whoever refreshes others will be refreshed"* (Acts 20:35, Proverbs 11:25).

Albert: Obscure Significance

Many noteworthy people work for the health of people at hospitals, like physicians, surgeons, nurses, and a polisher of shoes— polisher of shoes? Yes, a polisher of shoes was significant. He worked at a hospital shining shoes for twenty-eight years, making about ten thousand dollars a year. He worked at the Children's Hospital of Pittsburgh starting in 1981 and retiring in 2013. During those twenty-eight years, he received over 202,000 dollars in tips but didn't keep a penny for himself. Instead, he donated every dollar to the "Free Care Fund." That fund ensures that children who need medical care receive it whether their families can pay or not.

This man, Albert Lexie, passed away recently at the age of 76. He would get up at 5:50 every morning and would be at work by 7:25 each day for twenty-eight years. His purpose was not just to shine shoes but rather to donate every tip he received to benefit sick, uninsured children. The hospital's president said about Lexie that he was "a perfect example of how just small, incremental acts of kindness can have a significant impact over time."[78] Let's keep doing the small obscure acts of kindness too because they can make a difference in the lives of people! *"Always try to be kind to each other and to everyone else"* (1 Thessalonians 5:15).

Watch: "Pittsburgh Shoe shiner donates $200K in tips to Needy Children" https://www.youtube.com/watch?v=D4nFAjJy2f8

Unusual Resolutions

"Everyone has a future; some plan theirs." Some people make resolutions, but few keep them. Some research indicates that about 62% of people make New Year's resolutions, but only 8% achieve them. If people could achieve their resolutions, they would be very beneficial and meaningful like in spending less and saving more, staying fit and healthy, helping others and spending more time with family.

None of the examples mentioned are unusual. However, have you ever heard of a person making a New Year's Resolution to donate a kidney to an unknown person in need? That is not a normal resolution! When the need was noticed, she kept her resolution too.

David's kidneys had shut down; he was on kidney dialysis. The dialysis had started five years ago when he was only twenty-four. He wasn't handling his situation very well. He knew he was not in a good frame of mind and that his situation was tough, and getting tougher. He was on a donor's list, which doctors said could take years to find a match. Proverbs 18:14 was coming true in him. *"A man's spirit sustains him in sickness, but a crushed spirit who can bear?"*

He decided to try one more place, so he asked for help on Craigslist. Asking is the principle Jesus teaches on the "sermon on the mount" when he said, *"Ask and it will be given to you; seek and you will find; knock and the door will be opened to you. For everyone who asks receives; the one who seeks finds; and to the one who knocks, the door will be opened"* (Matthew 7:7-8). When David put an ad on Craigslist asking for a kidney, he got several responses. Most were foreign donors wanting money and help in immigrating to America, but one stood out.[79]

Jessica, the twenty-nine-year-old surgical nurse, responded. She was the one who had made the resolution she intended to keep. David, at first, thought her response was just another scam. Testing proved they were a match. On June 14, his situation improved as he received a kidney that changed his life. He does not look at Jessica as a fraud, but rather, he sees her as a "gift from God." Let's remember, we are to *"walk in the way of love"* (Ephesians 5:2). We are to *"always try to be kind to each other and to everyone else"* (1 Thessalonians 5:15). Kindness comes in many plans, as shown through Jessica.

Goodness in a 100-Year-Old

The day a woman turns 100, she is honored to throw the ceremonial pitch at a professional baseball game. She says she has waited 100 years to throw the pitch. "I never could have imagined celebrating a birthday like this, let alone my 100th," says Helen Kahan of St. Petersburg, Florida. We can understand how amazing this is once we realize she survived three Nazi concentration camps and escaped from a death march in Nazi-occupied Germany.

With a great depth of understanding and insight, she says the following: "I'm so grateful that I am here to tell my story and help the world remember why kindness and empathy are so important for us all." In the Holocaust, she lost her parents, sisters, brothers, and grandmothers." After experiencing such horrible circumstances, becoming bitter, resentful, and filled with hate would be easy. The 100-year-old Helen chose a different path, a path the proverb describes in this way. *"The path of the righteous is like the morning sun, shining ever brighter till the full light of day"* (Proverbs 4:18).

The Holocaust showed the worst of evil, but some people like Helen found a way to stay positive despite it. People describe her as a "sunny person." She lives her life with appreciation, being grateful for surviving even though so many others, including her family, didn't. She remembers growing up in a happy family. This is her advice for living a good life. "Be strong and help everybody." "Be **good** to people and just do the best you can do." Helen has been doing good since those terrible days of World War II. She married another Holocaust survivor, and they raised two daughters. Her family has expanded with five grandchildren and twelve great-grandchildren.[80]

Her words remind me of Paul's instructions. He encourages Titus, *"In everything set them an example by doing what is* **good***"* (Titus 2:7). Paul also writes this. *"Our people must learn to devote themselves to doing what is* **good***, in order to provide for urgent needs and not live unproductive lives"* (Titus 3:14). The Greek Lexicon on the word **good**—καλός kalos means "right or beautiful." People can do ugly, disgusting, hideous acts that are so cruel, but we need to see what is beautiful. Paul gives this instruction on how to overcome such things. *"Do not be overcome by evil, but overcome evil with good"* (Romans 12:21). Before that statement, he gives an example from the Proverbs. *"If your enemy is hungry, feed him; if he is thirsty, give him something to drink. In doing this, you will heap burning coals on his head."* Let's practice goodness and overcome evil!

Traveling and Helping

Traveling the road toward Boise, Idaho, a gust of wind caused the driver to over-compensate, lose control of the car and flip it off the road. The driver of a van behind that car saw all of this happen. At first, he only saw kicked-up dust, not knowing the car's condition. As the dust settled, he stopped and noticed the overturned car. He told the six others in the van to stay put until he could go and see the extent of the tragedy. He hoped he wouldn't see anything gruesome, and as he didn't, he called six youth football offensive linemen out of the van. They were thirteen or fourteen years old. To rescue the passenger, Alan Hardeman, they partially lifted the car. He had passed out in the crash, but "young voices" were trying to help wake him.[81]

His wife was still stuck behind the steering wheel. A second van soon arrived, loaded with more football players. This team had just won a California championship tournament. Their season was 11-0, but this rescue event gave these players an important perspective. One player took a video of the event. He thought it was amazing what they were able to do and did not want to imagine what would have happened if they had not been there to help.

Next, a dozen players lifted the car, and Alan's wife was rescued. Neither of them appeared to have severe injuries. A Deputy Sheriff was unable to arrive until about an hour after the accident. Alan Hardeman expressed his appreciation. He saw no hesitation to help from the team and did not know what they would have done without them!

A few days later, the team visited the home of the Hardeman's daughter where the couple was recovering. They came with flowers, cookies, and cards and presented them with a signed jersey and football. One player couldn't rescue them, but twelve could. Strength came with numbers along with the attitude to help! These players were practicing God's wisdom in helping the needy. *"Blessed is the one who is kind to the needy"* (Proverbs 14:21). The whole team was focused and ready to help. If we will walk with others, share information, and support them in the challenges they face, we too will be a helping team. *"Two are better than one, because they have a good return for their labor: If either of them falls down, one can help the other up. But pity anyone who falls and has no one to help them up"* (Ecclesiastes 4:9-10).

Watch: "Youth football team saves couple in overturned car" at https://www.youtube.com/watch?v=AmNbPKIACSU

40,000

What would you do with a ring you find while using a metal detector on a beach? A man found a ring on a beach near St. Augustine, Florida, south of Jacksonville. Next, his integrity or honesty is activated. *"The integrity of the upright guides them, but the unfaithful are destroyed by their duplicity"* (Proverbs 11:3). This man explains integrity with his actions! After he found the ring, he thought it might be worth two thousand dollars. Once he took it to a jeweler for evaluation, he was shocked that its estimated value is 40,000 dollars! "I couldn't believe it," he said. "That ring has been sitting in my scooter for almost a week."

Then what did he do? Instead of taking it to a resale store, he tried to find the owner by calling forty jewelry stores up and down the coast! Even though that did not seem to work, he still kept the ring. After two weeks, he received a call from an unidentified number. They tried calling him several times, but he wouldn't answer. Finally, he decided to answer as he thought this could be the ring's owner, and it was.

Back to the word *"integrity"*, that means *"being complete"* or *"finished."* The author of 1 Kings used the term to describe the temple. *"And he overlaid the whole house with gold, until all the house was **finished**. Also the whole altar that belonged to the inner* *sanctuary he overlaid with gold"* (1 Kings 6:22). Being *"finished"* meant the temple was complete.

Integrity also describes moral and ethical completeness or soundness. *"Keep your servant also from willful sins; may they not rule over me. Then I will be **blameless**, innocent of great transgression"* (Psalm 19:13). This was the soundness of Joseph Cook when he found the ring. He was blameless; he was a man of integrity. When a newsperson asked whether he thought about keeping it or selling it, he answered he never thought about selling it or saving it even for a minute. That action was never on his mind. Instead, he intended to return it to the owners, and that is what he did. He is a man of integrity and completeness. "They were pretty happy," he said. "The wife was on a FaceTime call, and she just said, I can't believe it, and then she just started crying." Not only did Joseph contribute to her happiness, but his own as well. *"A generous person will prosper; whoever refreshes others will be refreshed"* (Proverbs 11:25). He said, "It felt really good, I've returned sixty-thousand dollars of stuff this year, but nothing even close to this before." He refreshed the owner and himself by being generous. Let Joseph be our model.

The Story of Firefighters Saving a Man Who Becomes a Firefighter

Remember a time when you felt grateful for something that someone did for you! That "something" is usually meaningful and significant. When one person shared the details of what others did for him, he described them as life-changing for his life was literally saved. "That's not all they saved," he said. "They saved my family the pain of losing me. They saved my little sister's big brother. They saved me the time with my family that I would've never gotten." Does that sound significant? Does that sound meaningful? How was he saved?

Firefighters saved him. He was on the second floor of an apartment complex that was ablaze like a bonfire. This fire was huge! After climbing the ladder and going through the window a firefighter had found him unconscious. He awoke three days later in ICU at the hospital. Nurses told him what happened. He spent the next week in the hospital recovering. His story and the remembrance of what they had done for him motivated him.

Four years later a stranger arrived at the fire station for a "ride-along" (a program designed for observation of a day in the life of a firefighter). At first, no one recognized him until fifteen minutes later he told the major who he was—the person they carried out of an apartment fire four-years before and saved his life! They had given him a great desire! He desired to save others' lives! He had decided to earn his firefighter's degree.[82]

The Story of Zacchaeus

Two thousand years ago another man's life was saved. No one would have anything to do with him. He was an outcast because he was a hated tax collector. No one would expect the rabbi, the teacher, to go to his home and eat with him. His name was Zacchaeus and since he was so short, he climbed a sycamore-fig tree to see Jesus among the crowd. *"When Jesus reached the spot, he looked up and said to him, 'Zacchaeus, come down immediately. I must stay at your house today' So, he came down at once and welcomed him gladly."* Then we find him saying something very interesting. His life was being changed by Jesus. Jesus coming to his home was already motivating kindness in him. He said, *"Look, Lord! Here and now I give half of my possessions to the poor, and if I have cheated anybody out of anything, I will pay back four times the amount"* (Luke 19:5-6, 8). Zacchaeus was showing he was a changed man, a man of compassion. Jesus had saved this outcast's life. Would this be the "something" Zacchaeus could remember with gratitude? When we think back on events that others have done for us, it brings out the best in us. It happened to the man saved by firefighters and it happened to Zacchaeus. *"For the Son of Man came to seek and to save the lost"* (Luke 19:10).

Jesus had a reputation for being compassionate and kind toward people. He cared about people. When he looked at people, he pictured them as being harassed and helpless like sheep without a shepherd. He saw hurting people! *"He said to his disciples, 'The harvest is plentiful but the workers are few. Ask the Lord of the harvest, therefore, to send out workers into his harvest field'"* (Matthew 9:37-38.) He saw the need for more kind, compassionate workers!

The Story of the Apostle Paul

One man remembered a man who saved his life two thousand years ago, rescuing him from a destructive lifestyle. If this man could change from a vicious lifestyle to a lifestyle of gratitude, service, and love, so can anyone. He described himself as a persecutor, a violent man, and the worst of sinners. Why did he describe himself as a violent man? Hunting for people who were disciples of Jesus, forcing them to deny Jesus or face imprisonment or execution, is why he considered himself violent. He separated families with imprisonment or death when they refused to deny Jesus. He says, *"Many a time I went from one synagogue to another to have them punished, and I tried to force them to blaspheme. In my obsession against them, I even went to foreign cities to persecute them"* (Acts 26:11). Who or what could change such a vicious man?

The kindness and love he saw in a man who cared about people motivated him to live a life of love. He describes his new way of life with these words he wrote to a young man named Timothy. *"You, however, know all about my teaching, my way of life, my purpose, faith, patience, love, endurance, persecutions, sufferings"* (2 Timothy 3:10-11). His new life caused him to face persecution rather than be the perpetrator. Kindness has a strange response at times, like ugly violence, but usually appreciation. His lifestyle, in his words, *"In everything I did, I showed you that by this kind of hard work we must help the weak, remembering the words the Lord Jesus himself said: 'It is more blessed to give than to receive'"* (Acts 20:35).

The kindness and love of Jesus changed Paul's life! Paul writes, *"Christ Jesus came into the world to save sinners—of whom I am the worst"* (1 Timothy 1:15). He describes patience and kindness as attributes of love, which is what Jesus had for him (1 Corinthians 13:4). Jesus' love for him, his mercy, and compassion changed his life from violence to kindness (read Titus 3:4-5). Treating people as Jesus did was his desire. He wrote, *"Be imitators of me as I am of Christ"* (1 Corinthians 11:1). Paul describes Jesus' disciples as *"God's handiwork, created in Christ Jesus to do good works"* (Ephesians 2:10). Saved, or delivered from his life of violence and sin meant he writes being *"devoted to doing what is good"* (Titus 3:8). Grasping the depth of Jesus' love for him compelled him to live, not for himself, but for Jesus—to live a life of love (2 Corinthians 5:14, Ephesians 5:2).

Struck blind while hunting down disciples of Jesus to force them to deny their loyalty to Jesus or be imprisoned or even put to death gave him, in a sense, new life (Acts 26:11). He was on the road to Damascus when a bright light from heaven blinded him. Jesus spoke to him, saying, *"Saul, Saul, why do you persecute me?"* *"Who are you, Lord?" Saul asked. "I am Jesus, whom you are persecuting,"* he replied. *"Now get up and go into the city, and you will be told what you must do"* (Acts 9:4-6). So, he went to Damascus. Blind, praying and fasting for three days, Ananias, a disciple of Jesus, came to him and said, *"And now what are you waiting for? Get up, be baptized and wash your sins away, calling on his name"* (Acts 22:16). At that moment, he was saved, becoming a disciple of Jesus.

He could see again, but he saw life differently. He now had a new life. He was a new creation. *"If anyone is in Christ, the new creation has come: The old has gone, the new is here"* (2 Corinthians 5:17). All the havoc and harm he brought to people is now forgiven, washed away! He was a changed man. Instead of persecuting people, he began telling people how much Jesus loved them as he lived a life of love himself.

When he told people how to become compassionate, kind disciples of Jesus, he tied it directly to what Jesus had done for them. *"Or don't you know that all of us who were baptized into Christ Jesus were baptized into his death? We were therefore buried with him through baptism into death in order that, just as Christ was raised from the dead through the glory of the Father, we too may live a new life"* (Romans 6:3-4). And just how much does he say Jesus loves us? *"You see, at just the right time, when we were still powerless, Christ died for the ungodly. Very rarely will anyone die for a righteous person, though for a good person someone might possibly dare to die. But God demonstrates his own love for us in this: While we were still sinners, Christ died for us"* (Romans 5:6-8). A righteous person is just and fair, whereas a good person is just, fair, and generous. But Jesus died, demonstrating his love for the ungodly.

We are all in the ungodly category, yet Jesus was still willing to die for us. That makes us, in Jesus' view most valuable people! So, the apostle John writes, *"This is how we know what love is: Jesus Christ laid down his life for us"* (1 John 3:16). In summarizing Jesus' life, Peter said, *"he went around doing good"* (Acts 10:38). Paul was changed to do good, and let's do the same! Let's help people win a victory over diabetes!

Eyesight, Diabetic Retinopathy, and a Compassionate Doctor

This is an event I remember that made such a positive impact on my life. Thirty-seven years ago, as my wife and I and our two little boys were walking around a lake, I experienced a traumatic event. A dot appeared in my right eye. The dot kept growing. The beauty of the walkway and the lake were becoming a blur. By the time we got back to our car, I could barely see. I was experiencing a hemorrhage in the vitreous of my eye. We had just moved to a new state and town. I knew no doctor for support.

Fortunately, a new friend in our church informed me of a specialist — an endocrinologist — Dr. Richard Hellman (in 2007-2008, he was president of the American Association of Clinical

Endocrinologists). I saw him almost immediately. He then referred me to an ophthalmologist, Dr. Matthew Ziemianski. The hemorrhage was distressing enough, but add the shocking surprise that my health insurance company had just gone bankrupt made the situation an overwhelming burden! While sitting in the waiting room with my wife and two little boys, the doctor's nurse overheard a conversation I was having about my situation with another patient. She then informed the doctor.

So when I went into the doctor's office, he made a statement that I still get emotional about to this day, thirty-seven years later. He said his nurse had told him of my situation. Then he told me he would do laser treatment on my eyes without charge! He had seen me sitting in the waiting room with my wife and two little boys. I remember his words as if he spoke them yesterday: "Those boys need a father who can see." So, I'm going to do the surgeries without charge. He used the pan-retinal laser photocoagulation treatment in both eyes. When he said that, his words were the most meaningful and encouraging thing he could have said to me then. He did an excellent job with the laser treatment, helping me now have, thirty-seven years later, very good eyesight. His compassion and kindness were so significant that I was motivated to help others with support groups, diabetes educational seminars, and three books! Let's all be compassionate to others. We will then make a positive difference in their lives and ours! *"A generous person will prosper (be healthy); whoever refreshes others will be refreshed"* (Proverbs 11:25).

About the Authors

Ken Ellis is a survivor of diabetes for sixty-three years. During the fall of his first-grade year, he received the diagnosis of Type 1 Diabetes. For more than thirty years, he has facilitated hospital and community diabetes support groups, helping hundreds of people manage their diabetes in several states.

Ken has participated in the 50-year medalist research study and has been awarded the 50-Year Medal from the world-renowned Joslin Diabetes Center, which is affiliated with Harvard Medical School in Boston. This award represents his accomplishment in diabetes management for fifty years.

Deb Ellis is an administrative assistant. She is experienced in corporate, government, and school administration assistant responsibilities. More importantly, she is Ken's wife for almost fifty years, helping him with diabetes educational seminars, meal planning, and giving positive support for his diabetes management!

Ken's Education: Degree of Master of Science in Biblical Studies, Abilene Christian University, 1982

Contact: www.wisdomfordiabetes.org
Email: ken@wisdomfordiabetes.org

Bible Versions

Bibliography

Michael Bliss, **The Discovery of Insulin** (The University of Chicago Press, Chicago, 1982)

Dr. Sheri R. Colberg, **Diabetes and Keeping Fit** (by John Wiley & Sons, Inc., Hoboken, New Jersey, 2018)

Ken Ellis, **7 Biblical Ways for Healthy Living**

Ken Ellis, **The Way of Wisdom for Diabetes**

Robert A. Emmons, Ph.D., **Thanks! How Practicing Gratitude Can Make You Happier** (Houghton Mifflin Company, New York, 2007)

Dr. Jason Fung, **Diabetes Code** (Greystone Books Ltd., 2018)

Jessie Inchauspe**, Glucose Revolution:** The Life-Changing Power of Balancing Your Blood Sugar (Simon Element, New York, 2022)

Jordin Ruben and Dr. Josh Axe, **Essential Fasting:** 12 Benefits of Intermittent Fasting (DESTINY IMAGE® PUBLISHERS, INC., 2020).

Endnotes

1   Texas Police Make Odd Withdrawal from ATM: A Man Who
    Was Trapped Inside, Colin Dwyer, https://www.npr.org/
    sections/thetwo-way/2017/07/13/537043822/texas-
    police-make-odd-withdrawal-from-atm-a-man-who-was-
    trapped-inside (Accessed August 2023)

2   Richard Beaser, MD, ed., Joslin Diabetes Deskbook: A
    Guide for Primary Care Providers (Boston: Joslin Diabetes
    Center, 2014), 4, 5.

3   Dan J. Weinert, Nutrition and muscle protein synthesis: a
    descriptive review (August 2009) https://www.ncbi.nlm.
    nih.gov/pmc/articles/PMC2732256/ (Accessed August
    2023).

4   Jason Fung, MD, The Diabetes Code: Prevent and Reverse
    Type 2 Diabetes Naturally (Greystone Books Ltd., 2018),
    80.

5   Matthew T. Draelos, MD, Health Tips https://www.
    draelosmetabolic.com/dr-draelos-health-tips (Accessed
    March 2019).

6   Incretin Hormone, Diabetes Self-management, (March 13, 2009) https://www.diabetesselfmanagement.com/diabetes-resources/definitions/incretin-hormone/ (Accessed March 2019).

7   Jennie Brand-Miller, PhD, Kaye Foster-Powell, and Rick Mendosa, What Makes My Blood Glucose Go Up . . . and Down?: And 101 Other Frequently Asked Questions About Your Blood Glucose Levels (New York: Marlowe & Company, 2003), 173-182.

8   Richard Beaser, MD, ed., Joslin Diabetes Deskbook: A Guide for Primary Care Providers (Boston: Joslin Diabetes Center, 2014), 112.

9   Robert A. Emmons, Thanks: How Practicing Gratitude Can Make You Happier (New York: Houghton Mifflin Company, 2007), 27, 32–33.

10   Rob Thompson M.D. and Dana Carpender, The Insulin Resistance Solution: Reverse Pre-Diabetes, Repair Your Metabolism, Shed Belly Fat, Prevent Diabetes

11   Sheri R. Colberg, Diabetes and Keeping Fit For Dummies (pp. 189-190). Wiley. Kindle Edition.

12   Exercise intensity: How to measure it, https://www.mayoclinic.org/healthy-lifestyle/fitness/in-depth/exercise-intensity/art-20046887 (Accessed July 2019).

13   Standing for healthier lives—literally, Francisco Lopez-Jimenez, MD, Mayo Clinic. https://academic.oup.com/eurheartj/article/36/39/2650/2398350 (Accessed May 2018).

14   Researchers say to stand up, sit less and move more. Carolina Storrs, CNN August 6, 2015, http://www.cnn.com/2015/08/06/health/how-to-move-more/index.html (Accessed May 2018).

15   Sheri R. Colberg, Diabetes and Keeping Fit For Dummies (pp. 189-190). Wiley. Kindle Edition.

16   'I Have Terminal Brain Cancer. I Just Did An Ironman To Inspire My 5-Year-Old,' Jenny Haward, https://www.newsweek.com/i-have-terminal-brain-cancer-i-just-did-ironman-inspire-daughter-1538800 (Accessed August, 2023).

17   Walter Willett, MD, Eat, Drink, and Weigh Less: A Flexible and Delicious Way to Shrink your Waist Without Going Hungry (New York: Tante Malka, Inc., 2006), 67.

18   Drinking Water May Cut Risk of High Blood Sugar, Charlene Laino, http://diabetes.webmd.com/news/20110630/drinking-water-may-cut-risk-of-high-blood-sugar (Accessed March 12, 2018).

19   Barbara Rolls, Ph.D., The Volumetrics Eating Plan: Techniques and Recipes for Feeling Full on Fewer Calories (New York: HarperCollins Publishers, 2005), 10.

20   Artificial sweeteners: sugar-free, but at what cost? Holly Strawbridge https://www.health.harvard.edu/blog/artificial-sweeteners-sugar-free-but-at-what-cost-2017165030 (Accessed March 16, 2018).

21   Urine Color, Mayo Clinic Staff, https://www.mayoclinic.org/diseases-conditions/urine-color/symptoms-causes/syc-20367333 (Accessed March 12, 2018)

22 Water and Stress Reduction: Sipping Stress Away, Gina Shaw, http://www.webmd.com/diet/features/water-stress-reduction (Accessed March 12, 2018).

23 Robert K. Cooper, Ph.D., Flip the Switch Lose the Weight: Proven Strategies to Fuel Your Metabolism & Burn Fat 24 Hours a Day (New York: Rodale Inc., 2005), 78-79.

24 Brian Wansink, Ph.D., Mindless Eating: Why We Eat More Than We Think (New York: Bantam Dell, 2006), 189.

25 Dr. Jason Fung. The Diabetes Code: 2 (The Code Series) (p. 219). Greystone Books. Kindle Edition.

26 Mark Ehrman and Sara Mednick, Take a Nap! Change Your Life. (pp. 23-28). Workman Publishing Company May 2018. Kindle Edition.

27 The Health Benefits of Napping: Resting Can Help Reduce Stress and Protect Immune System, Lecia Bushak, Medical Daily, February 10, 2015, http://www.medicaldaily.com/health-benefits-napping-resting-can-help-reduce-stress-and-protect-immune-system-321580 (Accessed August 2019).

28 How to get the most out of napping, Micah Dorfner, https://newsnetwork.mayoclinic.org/discussion/how-to-get-the-most-out-of-napping/ March 28, 2018 (Accessed August 2019).

29 Jessie Inchauspe, Glucose Revolution: The Life-Changing Power of Balancing Your Blood Sugar (p. 92). S&S/Simon Element. Kindle Edition.

30 Broccoli Nutrition Helps Battle Cancer, Osteoporosis & Weight Gain, Jillian Levy, CHHC October 3, 2022, https://draxe.com/nutrition/broccoli-nutrition/

31   Break the Cycle of Yo-Yo Dieting, Jennifer Hubert, DO
      January 9, 2018 https://blog.providence.org/healthcalling/
      break-the-cycle-of-yo-yo-dieting

32   Rob Thompson, M.D., and Dana Carpender. The Insulin
      Resistance Solution: Reverse Pre-Diabetes, Repair Your
      Metabolism, Shed Belly Fat, Prevent Diabetes (p. 62).
      Quarto Publishing Group USA. Kindle Edition.

33   Ibid (p. 62).

34   Remembering Ida Keeling, Who Set Track Records into
      Her 100s, Nadia Neophytou Sept 15, 2021 (Accessed
      August 2023).

35   Osama Hamdy and Sheri R. Colberg, Sheri R, The Diabetes
      Breakthrough: Based on a Scientifically Proven Plan to
      Lose Weight and Cut Medications (Kindle Location 2950).
      Harlequin. Kindle Edition.

36   Ozempic for Weight Loss: How Does It Work and Who Can
      Use It?, Alyssa Billingsley, PharmD and Christina Aungst,
      PharmD, Updated on April 26, 2023

37   Mounjaro More Effective Than Ozempic for Weight Loss,
      New Research Shows, Victoria Stokes, August 2, 2023

38   Could the Timing of When You Eat, Be Just as Important
      as What You Eat? Science Daily, January 29, 2013,
      Source: Brigham and Women's Hospital http://www.
      sciencedaily.com/releases/2013/01/130129080620.htm
      (Accessed August 2019)

39 Time-restricted feeding study shows promise in helping people shed body fat, Adam Pope, January 09, 2017, https://www.uab.edu/news/health/item/7869-time-restricted-feeding-study-shows-promise-in-helping-people-shed-body-fat (Accessed August 2019).

40 Stages of Fasting by Hour and Fat Burning Stage Fasting, June 5, 2022, https://kompanionapp.com/en/fasting-fat-burning-stage/

41 How Much Sleep Do I Need?, https://www.cdc.gov/sleep/about_sleep/how_much_sleep.html (Accessed August 2019).

42 How Much Sleep Do Fitbit Users Really Get? A New Study Finds Out, Danielle Kosecki, June 29, 2017, https://blog.fitbit.com/sleep-study/ (Accessed August 2019).

43 Drowsy Driving: Asleep at the Wheel, https://www.cdc.gov/features/dsdrowsydriving/index.html (Accessed August 2019).

44 Michael Breus. The Sleep Doctor's Diet Plan: Simple Rules for Losing Weight While You Sleep (p. 8). Potter/Ten Speed/Harmony/Rodale. Kindle Edition.

45 Sleep and Metabolism: An Overview, 2010, https://www.ncbi.nlm.nih.gov/pmc/articles/PMC2929498/ (Accessed August 2019)

46 Breus, 9-10.

47 Breus, 44.

48 Sleep and Metabolism: An Overview, Int J Endocrinol. 2010. https://www.ncbi.nlm.nih.gov/pmc/articles/PMC2929498/ (Accessed August 2019).

49 Breus, 28-29.

50   Maximising Your Melatonin, https://
instituteofhealthsciences.com/maximising-your-melatonin/
(Accessed August 2019).

51   Melatonin, https://www.webmd.com/vitamins/ai/
ingredientmono-940/melatonin (Accessed August 2019).

52   Top 20 Ways to Fall Asleep Fast! Dr. Josh Axe, https://
draxe.com/cant-sleep/ (Accessed August 2019).

53   Robert A. Emmons, Thanks: How Practicing Gratitude Can
Make You Happier (New York: Houghton Mifflin Company,
2007), 27. Emmons, 32–33.

54   Stephen Post, Why Good Things Happen to Good People:
The Exciting New Research That Proves the Link Between
Doing Good and Living a Longer, Healthier, Happier Life
(New York: Broadway Books, 2007), 28, 30.

55   Personal Accounts of the Negative and Adaptive
Psychosocial Experiences of People With Diabetes in the
Second Diabetes Attitudes, Wishes and Needs (DAWN2)
Study, Heather L. Stuckey,   Diabetes Care September,
2014 http://care.diabetesjournals.org/content/37/9/2466
(Accessed August 2019).

56   Richard Beaser, MD, ed., Joslin Diabetes Deskbook: A
Guide for Primary Care Providers (Boston: Joslin Diabetes
Center, 2014), 437-440.

57   John Walsh, PA, CDE, Using Insulin: Everything You Need
for Success with Insulin (San Diego: Torrey Pines Press,
2003), 220.

58 Loneliness is universal: Boca students' message that
    nobody should eat alone is heard worldwide, https://
    www.sun-sentinel.com/local/broward/fl-boca-raton-we-
    dine-together-goes-viral-20170417-story.html (Accessed
    August 2019).
59 A Bike Accident Left This ER Doctor Paralyzed.
    Now He's Back At Work, Chris Bentley, and Jeremy
    Hobson, (June 06, 2018), https://www.wbur.org/
    hereandnow/2018/06/06/doctor-paralyzed-mayo-clinic
    (Accessed March 2019).
60 US man clings to glider after taking off unsecured to craft,
    Bryce Luff, PerthNow, (November 27, 2018) https://www.
    perthnow.com.au/news/europe/us-man-clings-to-glider-
    after-taking-off-unsecured-to-craft-ng-b881033549z
    (Accessed March 2019).
61 Police officer stuck behind a tortoise posts video
    of his encounter https://www.youtube.com/
    watch?v=dUEz6AmUPPQ
62 Chris Feudtner, M.D., Bittersweet: Diabetes, Insulin, and
    the Transformation of Illness (Chapel Hill: The University
    of North Carolina Press, 2003), 52.
63 Michael Bliss, The Making of Modern Medicine: Turning
    Points in the Treatment of Disease (Chicago: The
    University of Chicago Press, 2011), 76.
64 Bliss, 76.
65 David O. Woodbury, "Please Save My Son" Reader's
    Digest, (volume 82, number 490, February, 1963), 157-
    162.

66   "Miracle Boy" Wakes From Coma Day Before Parents Pull The Plug On Life Support, May 7, 2018, https://alt1037dfw. radio.com/blogs/miracle-boy-wakes-coma-day-parents-pull-plug-life-support (Accessed August 2019).

67   Teen heart transplant patient finds miracle wrapped in delay, August 29, 2014, https://www.khou.com/article/ news/health/teen-heart-transplant-patient-finds-miracle-wrapped-in-delay/259142526 (Accessed August 2019).

68   Henry Dolger, M.D. and Bernard Seeman, How to Live with Diabetes (New York: Pyramid Books, 1958), 103.

69   Dolger, 84.

70   Woman Is Brought To Tears By Thank You Note After Act Of Kindness In Grocery Store, January 11, 2019, https:// www.sunnyskyz.com/good-news/3170/Woman-Is-Brought-To-Tears-By-Thank-You-Note-After-Act-Of-Kindness-In-Grocery-Store (Accessed August 2019).

71   A soldier says a stranger's Christmas card got him through Vietnam. He just met the sender, November 17, 2018, https://www.wivb.com/news/national/a-soldier-says-a-strangers-christmas-card-got-him-through-vietnam-he-just-met-the-sender/ (Accessed August 2019).

72   'Selfless' Patient Able to Continue Helping Others After Transplant, April 12, https://intheloop.mayoclinic. org/2018/04/12/selfless-patient-able-to-continue-helping-others-after-transplant/ (Accessed August 2019).

73   Homeless man finds $17,000, gives it to food bank, December 5, 2018, https://wgntv.com/2018/12/05/ homeless-man-finds-17000-gives-it-to-food-bank/ (Accessed August 2019).

74   Richard Jackson, MD, and Amy Tenderich, Know Your Numbers, Outlive Your Diabetes: Five Essential Health Factors You Can Master to Enjoy a Long and Healthy Life (New York: Marlowe & Company, 2007), 104, 107.

75   A father and his sons cut wood to fill 80 trucks. Then they brought it to homes that needed heat, Caitlin Huson, December 21, 2018, https://www.washingtonpost.com/lifestyle/2018/12/21/father-his-sons-cut-wood-fill-trucks-then-they-brought-it-homes-that-needed-heat/?noredirect=on (Accessed August 2019).

76   107-Year-Old Is The World's Oldest Barber And He's Still Cutting Hair Full Time, October 14, 2018, https://www.sunnyskyz.com/good-news/3040/107-Year-Old-Is-The-World-039-s-Oldest-Barber-And-He-039-s-Still-Cutting-Hair-Full-Time (Accessed August 2019).

77   99-year-old man walks 6 miles a day to visit his wife in the hospital, proving true love does exist, August 31, 2018, https://www.cbsnews.com/news/99-year-old-man-luther-younger-walks-six-miles-a-day-to-visit-his-wife-in-the-hospital-rochester-new-york/ (Accessed August 2019).

78   Albert Lexie, the shoe-shiner who donated $200K to UPMC Children's Hospital, has died, Bob Batz Jr. Pittsburgh Post-Gazette, October 16, 2018, https://www.post-gazette.com/news/obituaries/2018/10/16/albert-lexie-children-s-hospital-pittsburgh-shoe-shiner-monessen-obituary-foundation/stories/201810160158 (Accessed August 2019).

79   Woman's New Year's Resolution Saves A Stranger's
     Life, June 14, 2018, https://www.sunnyskyz.com/good-
     news/2855/Woman-039-s-New-Year-039-s-Resolution-
     Saves-A-Stranger-039-s-Life (Accessed August 2019).

80   Florida woman who survived Holocaust turns 100, throws
     first pitch at Yankees-Rays game: 'Really wonderfull,'
     Gretchen Eichenberg Fox News, May 8, 2023, https://
     www.foxnews.com/lifestyle/florida-woman-survived-
     holocaust-turns-100-throws-first-pitch-yankees-rays-
     game-really-wonderful

81   Boise youth football team meets with couple they
     helped rescue from overturned car, Michael Katz, Idaho
     Statesman, May 30 and June 1, 2018, https://www.
     idahostatesman.com/latest-news/article212236279.html
     (Accessed August 2019).

82   Metro Rescue Victim To Become Firefighter, Christy
     Lewis, Oklahoma City News9, February 23, 2018, http://
     www.news9.com/story/37580818/metro-rescue-victim-to-
     become-firefighter (Accessed August 2019).

Printed in Great Britain
by Amazon

30819621R00099